INTENSIVE CARE

The publisher gratefully acknowledges the generous contribution to this book provided by Orville and Ellina Golub.

INTENSIVE CARE

A Doctor's Journal

JOHN F. MURRAY, M.D.

University of California Press

Berkeley · Los Angeles · London

University of California Press
Berkeley and Los Angeles, California

University of California Press, Ltd.
London, England

© 2000 by the Regents of the University of California

Library of Congress Cataloging-in-Publication Data

Murray, John F. (John Frederic), 1927–
Intensive care : a doctor's journal / John F. Murray.
    p.   cm.
    Includes bibliographical references and index.
    ISBN 0-520-22089-7 (cloth : alk.)
    1. Critical care units—Anecdotes.   2. Critical care medi-
cine—Anecdotes.   I. Title.
RA975.5.I56 M87   2000
362.1'74—dc21   99-056892

Manufactured in the United States of America

09 08 07 06 05 04 03 02 01 00
10 9 8 7 6 5 4 3 2 1

The paper used in this publication meets the minimum
requirements of ANSI/NISO Z39.48-1992 (R 1997)
(Permanence of Paper). ∞

To Dinny, with love and thanks

CONTENTS

Prologue · *ix*

Day 1 *Thursday* · *1*

Day 2 *Friday* · *18*

Day 3 *Saturday* · *28*

Day 4 *Sunday* · *36*

Day 5 *Monday* · *48*

Day 6 *Tuesday* · *59*

Day 7 *Wednesday* · *68*

Day 8 *Thursday* · *79*

Day 9 *Friday* · *92*

Day 10 *Saturday* · *101*

Day 11 *Sunday* · *115*

Day 12 *Monday* · *125*

Day 13 *Tuesday* · *132*

Day 14 *Wednesday* · *141*

Day 15 *Thursday* · *151*

Day 16 *Friday* · *166*

Day 17 *Saturday* · *175*

Day 18 *Sunday* · *181*

Day 19 *Monday* · *191*

Day 20 *Tuesday* · *201*

Day 21 *Wednesday* · *212*

Day 22 *Thursday* · *218*

Day 23 *Friday* · *226*

Day 24 *Saturday* · *231*

Day 25 *Sunday* · *238*

Day 26 *Monday* · *244*

Day 27 *Tuesday* · *251*

Day 28 *Wednesday* · *259*

Epilogue · *267*

Notes · *277*

Acknowledgments · *283*

Index · *285*

PROLOGUE An unseen hand flings open the door to the intensive care unit. Then appears the back of a woman wearing a green scrub suit. She has a stethoscope draped around her neck—probably a medical resident. At her side is another woman in green, who helps her pull a bed in from the corridor by wrenching one end through the ICU door, which a nurse runs over to hold open. The other end of the bed is simultaneously pushed and guided by a young man who is shouting directions. He is flanked by a respiratory therapist doing his best to help push by leaning on the headboard, while both his hands are occupied with the repetitive squeezing of a melon-sized elastic bag, which fills automatically with oxygen from the green cylinder attached to the front of the bed.

From under a sheet and rumpled blanket extend the head and naked upper torso of a nearly bald man, perhaps in his forties or fifties, with a grizzled face, twisted nose, and cauliflower ears. Instead of a neck, huge muscles flare out from just below his ears to the tips of powerfully broad shoulders. He must once have been tremendously strong, maybe a professional football player or wrestler. But now his skin is sallow and his lips are ominously dusky. He seems lifeless except for the slow, deep rise and fall of his chest under the bedclothes as the therapist compresses the bag to force oxygen into the man's lungs through a clear plastic tube that protrudes from his mouth. A chrome yellow box—a portable unit for monitoring the heart and shocking it back to life if it stops—lies on the bed. The wires that attach the instrument to the patient's chest are out of sight, but each heartbeat is announced by a high-pitched ping. The accompanying electrocardiographic wave form is traced on a small screen for his guardians to observe.

While this improvised cortege negotiates its way through the door, the head nurse calls, "Room Three," and hurries ahead to clear the corridor of chairs, computers on pedestals, and other equipment. Inside Room Three another respiratory therapist waits with a ventilator, a life-preserving breathing machine that will automatically stuff oxygen into the patient's lungs. While he was in the emergency department, two slender plastic tubes, "cannulas," were inserted into the patient's veins, one in each arm, and a larger rubber catheter was implanted in his bladder. Once in the unit, a third and fourth cannula are added, one, in a vein, to provide extra access to the patient's bloodstream for medications and one, in an artery, to monitor his blood pressure. The patient appears tethered by the cat's cradle of tubes emerging from plastic bags that hang from stainless steel poles surrounding his bedside; appended pumps control the flow of fluids and medications into his body. A calibrated plastic bag, hanging empty, will collect urine once his beleaguered kidneys recover enough to produce some. Wires sprout from his chest, where small patches of hair have been shaved for electrodes to be securely glued, and they all converge at a large television monitor mounted on the wall. A clothespin-like device, an oximeter, is clamped on his index finger to measure the level of oxygen circulating in his blood; its electrical connection also leads to the television set.

The screen displays numbers that register the patient's moment-to-moment heart rate, blood pressure, and level of oxygenation, as well as continuous tracings of his electrocardiogram, arterial pressure, and oximeter waveforms. Alarms are set to emit a particular identifying squeak, beep, or ring should a vital physiologic function deteriorate further. Apart from the flashing signals that his heart is beating and his blood pressure exists, propped up by powerful drugs, there are no signs of life. The rhythmic movements of his chest are an illusion created by the breathing machine that pumps in oxygen-enriched fresh air—no matter what.

So far so good. Everything is proceeding according to the formula of the medical dramas on television. But here, clinical reality and not television fiction determines the outcome. Whether the as yet unnamed patient, barely clinging to life, will leave the unit alive in the bed he now occupies, escorted by one of his cheerful nurses to a medical ward for further treatment, or whether his enshrouded corpse, perhaps still-unidentified, will leave on a gurney pushed by a dour morgue attendant, depends on how fast and accurately his physicians can diagnose and treat the cause of this catastrophe, and on how well his nurses anticipate and respond to the perilous events that will almost surely complicate the next few hours and days. This is what intensive care units (ICUs) are for, and it is what this book is about: how doctors and nurses make decisions concerning such urgent medical problems.

Ordinary patients are not cared for in ICUs. These select facilities are reserved for desperately sick patients, those who are likely to die without specialized medical attention, like the profoundly ill man just described. The use of ICUs to care for critically ill patients is a new but well-established and growing branch of medicine. The chief purpose of this book is to inform people about what really goes on in ICUs: who gets admitted, how extraordinarily ill patients are treated, and what happens to them. Few have this information, but it concerns everyone. We do not know exactly how many of us will require intensive care during our lifetimes, but perhaps fifteen to twenty percent of all hospitalized patients are now treated in an intensive care or coronary care unit (an ICU sibling dedicated to patients with heart disease) for some portion of each hospital stay.[1] If you consider the number of times a person growing older is likely to be hospitalized, this adds up to a lot of people. The odds strongly favor the possibility that an ICU will become a temporary home and a critical link to life for you or a family member.

Lives are indeed saved in the ICU; that is always the goal, and those of us who work there are good at achieving it. But the other side of the coin is that sometimes even highly sophisticated expert care doesn't work out as planned—patients die. One of the lessons of this book is that death is an ever-present part of the ICU story. Despite our mastery of medical science and technology, ICU doctors do not always succeed. Another lesson is that death is not a correctable biological condition— it is everyone's ultimate destiny. Finding that elusive boundary between extending life when there is a chance for more and allowing death when hope has truly gone is seldom easy, yet we undertake that search nearly every day. The reader will learn from actual medical histories that in the ICU we have the power either to delay or to accelerate the course of dying. My own view is—and you will see why as you read further—that the current decision-making process can and should be improved. Occasionally, a patient's treatment is sufficiently drawn out and degrading to warrant being termed "a managed death."[2] Sometimes treatments are given because they are technically possible, not because they are what patients necessarily want or need. Medicine relies heavily on the ICU's high-tech, high-cost ability to prolong life, but sometimes, despite our best intentions, intensive care lapses into the inhumane.

All this will be apparent during the four weeks we make daily ward rounds together in the medical ICU at San Francisco General Hospital (SFGH). My formal role there is that of "attending physician," the person who has final authority over all matters concerning the patients, and who is legally and morally responsible for everything that occurs during these four weeks. We will be joined in these regular tours by the usual entourage of residents in medicine, young physicians training to be specialists in internal medicine, and by medical students, generally even younger men and women in their last years of medical school. You will meet the patients as I meet them, one by one, as their histories are told to me by the residents and students assigned to care for them. SFGH is a "teaching hospital" and plays a key role in the University of California San Francisco (UCSF) Medical School teaching program. Thus, part of my responsibility as a member of the faculty of UCSF is to serve as ICU teacher-of-the-month for the residents and students who accompany me as we go from patient to patient, assessing their medical condition and deciding what to do next.

Our ICU is livelier than many because we serve a medical community in a city known for its unusual mix of inhabitants. Like many city and county hospitals, SFGH is the main facility for the city's socioeconomically disadvantaged, and now we have a large number of people with HIV infection as well. Kindred institutions are Bellevue Hospital in New York City, Cook County Hospital in Chicago, Charity Hospital in New Orleans, and Harborview Hospital in Seattle—to mention only a few of the most prominent—all of which provide vital services to patients who, for one reason or another, are not welcome in private hospitals. Because our patients and their illnesses differ a bit from those in units elsewhere, our ICU is not identical in every way to all the others. Nevertheless, an ICU is an ICU, and there are unquestionably more similarities than differences among the approximately six thousand acute care units in the United States.

For SFGH, the four-week period I have recorded here was ordinary in most respects: in the number of admissions and deaths; in the kinds of medical disorders and their severity; in the range of social and ethical problems. A close look at these twenty-eight days, then, offers a reasonable overview of what intensive care is meant to accomplish, how the system operates, and what obstacles can encumber the rescue of desperately ill people clinging to life or unreasonably torment people who are bound to die.

These are my notes (set in italicized type) more or less as I wrote them down in the patients' medical records at the time, along with my later reflections (set in regular type) about some of the patients whose individual stories went unappreciated in the urgency of the days we were trying to keep them alive and from whom we have much to learn about this difficult specialty. It may be that you will think you recognize some patients, perhaps as relatives or friends, even as yourself. Numerous people become afflicted with exactly the same diseases, ones diagnosed according to a typical constellation of clinical features, x-ray abnormalities, and laboratory findings. Thus, similarities are sure to occur among the many patients with the same disease. Although events and descriptions in this book come from true clinical situations, to protect the privacy of the particular patients who are depicted, certain identifying information has been altered or deleted.

DAY	
1	*Thursday*

I walked onto the ICU a little before 8:00 A.M. to find three third-year medical residents— Dr. Ella Andrews, Dr. James Shotinger, and Dr. Ian Trent-Johnson—waiting for me. Each had a big smile. They had arrived early to familiarize themselves with our patients and already knew a lot about them. Their smiles were not only welcoming but inquiring. We were all going to spend the next four weeks together, and they were curious to see how well I would help them handle the formidable problems that lay ahead of us: would I be an aid or an obstacle, a rabid interventionist or a do-nothing conservative, a stickler or a laissez-faire leader? Could I teach? Now in the last year of medical residency, they had learned that much of their training in internal medicine is subject to variations in attending physicians' style and competence.

While they were wondering about me, I was scrutinizing them. Depending on their clinical abilities and willingness to work hard, the four weeks I would spend in the units and my level of anxiety during our rotation together would be either manageable or exceedingly uncomfortable. I would be depending on them, and on a number of other personnel as well, to carry out the plans we had agreed on during rounds, to show good judgment in dealing with new patients and with matters we had not discussed, and to contact me if something came up that they were uncertain about. Each patient admitted to SFGH with a medical problem is assigned to the care of a housestaff team; the leader of the team is a second-year resident who supervises two first-year residents and, usually, one or two medical students. The members of this team follow their patients throughout their stay in the hospital, wherever they go, including the ICU, where there is another layer of medical supervision, the third-year residents who work with me. Our resident on call today, attractive and talkative Ella Andrews, moved quickly to the nearest phone to page the first of the teams who would come to tell us about their new patient. That is when our month in the ICU begins.

Her family had decided that Jisoo Hong should die, but she was not allowed to. Mrs. Hong is a seventy-six-year-old Korean-speaking woman with multiple chronic medical problems, whose mind is lost forever behind a shroud of dementia. Her mental blankness is presumably the result of numerous strokes; she has no idea who or where she is, she cannot talk or communicate in any fashion, and she is totally blind. She also has serious heart disease, which required surgical implantation of an electronic pacemaker to sustain a regular heartbeat, and she suffers from diabetes mellitus ("sugar" diabetes), which necessitates insulin every day. As the admitting first-year resident tells us, because of the severity and irreversibility of her problems, the family decided several months ago that if a medical catastrophe were to occur—and one was inevitable—she should be allowed to die peacefully and should not be resuscitated if her heart stopped. Nor should she have a painful tube inserted through her mouth or nose and fastened in her windpipe—a procedure called intubation that enables a ventilator to assist someone's breathing.

Intubation is a common and crucial ICU maneuver. But in people who are awake, intubation is extremely disagreeable and must be performed using local anesthetics to block the powerful cough-and-gag reflexes triggered by the procedure. Imagine having a one-foot-long plastic tube thicker than your index finger scrape along the back of your throat, force its way between your vocal cords, and finally be fixed within your windpipe by a balloon inflated near the tip. Painful sensations inevitably return when the anesthesia wears off and the reflexes wake up. When patients cannot breathe by themselves or cough to prevent food and liquids from entering their windpipes, intubation *must* be done to save their lives; but just as soon as it is safe, we take the tube out because most patients fear and hate it. Many of the decisions we have to make are dictated by this dreaded but often necessary tube.

Intubating a patient like Mrs. Hong is inhumane unless there are clinical rewards to offset the torment and numerous potential complications. We agree completely with her own family's and physician's decision not to intubate her. But here she is—intubated!

At home two days before, Mrs. Hong had trouble breathing during the night. Yesterday morning she developed a fever, and later in the day her unmarried niece, who has devoted the last five years to caring for her aunt, finally panicked and called 9 1 1. The ambulance crew responded quickly and found Mrs. Hong laboring to breathe, with frothy secretions gurgling in her throat, a sign Hippocrates, the Father of Medicine, recognized more than two thousand years ago and called the "death rattle." But the paramedics cleaned her air passages with suction and brought Mrs. Hong to SFGH, where the physicians in the emergency department, in total ignorance of the previous decision not to intubate, acted on the urgent medical demands of the moment and put a tube in her windpipe. Then they sent her to us in the ICU for machine-supported breathing. They also began antibiotic treatment for pneumonia—clearly the cause of her respiratory distress.

By the time I see her this morning, all this critical background information has been uncovered. The first-year resident who called her private physician, Dr. Ira Constant, in the middle of the night, reported sheepishly, "He shrieked at me."

"She's what? Intubated! You guys are out of your minds," Dr. Constant had

shouted. "Do you know how many hours I spent persuading her family she should NOT be intubated? Now you've screwed it all up." Dr. Constant's distress is justified. After his considerable efforts to spare Mrs. Hong the misery of intubation, that is exactly what has been inflicted on her.

Pneumonia—what Sir William Osler, one of the demigods of early twentieth-century medicine, called "the old person's friend"—was trying to put an easy end to a life that had no positive quality except in the mind of her niece, a reclusive woman in her fifties who was totally absorbed in caring for her aunt and could not allow her to die quietly at home—even though the legally responsible members of the family had decided that was the best possible course. The niece called the paramedical personnel, who did what they are trained to do expertly: they saved her aunt's life. So did the physicians in the emergency service. Everything unfolds fast in these situations, and there is little opportunity to derail the process. Dr. Constant is right. We had screwed it up, albeit inadvertently.

In 1991 California instituted a system for staving off inadvisable resuscitations, including intubation such as Jisoo Hong had, or efforts to revive an impotent heart, *before* patients arrive at the hospital and their medical records become available. A similar mechanism had long existed for patients already hospitalized. Together, patients or their surrogates and physicians can fill out and sign a special prehospital Do Not Resuscitate (DNR) form that orders emergency medical service (EMS) personnel to forego resuscitation attempts if the patient's heart stops or breathing ceases. But even this simple process does not always work: many physicians—like Dr. Constant, as it turned out—do not know about it, and even if the form is filled out, it has to be shown to the right person in time to prevent or abort action. It is hard to imagine Mrs. Hong's niece waving such an order in front of the paramedics as they were suctioning her aunt's throat and windpipe. Had Mrs. Hong been wearing one of the available bracelets or neck medallions inscribed with the words "DO NOT RESUSCITATE—EMS," her niece's desire to override the family's intentions would have been thwarted. This alerting system, alas, is neither automatic nor foolproof; the bracelet or medallion must be obtained separately and paid for, after the form is completed, and then worn at all times.

Fortunately, the treatment Mrs. Hong had received for her pneumonia had helped enough that we could begin to take her off the ventilator. That afternoon, we disconnected it and took the tube out of her windpipe, and in the evening we moved her out of the ICU and into a regular ward. At no time did she respond when we talked to her, even when she was spoken to in Korean by one of SFGH's team of masterly interpreters, who among them know virtually every language and dialect. She just moaned and writhed intermittently, and looked tortured. Five days later when we heard she had gone home with her niece, I could only shrug helplessly, without any feeling of relief, knowing what was in store for her. Some other crisis was bound to occur, and I was certain that her niece's pitiful struggles to keep Mrs. Hong alive would add more misery to an already wretched existence.

Now we visit Charlotte Atkinson, a thirty-two-year-old part-time receptionist who came to SFGH three days ago after vomiting a large amount of bright red blood. She has severe bulimia, which is characterized by a preoccupation with weight and intense guilt about episodes of perceived overeating; these, in turn, are assuaged by purging or by self-induced vomiting. Her doctors learned that her habit of making herself vomit each time she ate had begun while she was about twenty years old and training to be a champion middle-distance runner. Professional running is associated with a high risk of eating disturbances, including bulimia, and other psychiatric complications that involve pushing body and mind past normal limits. She had won several races, but after she failed to qualify for the United States Olympic Team, she stopped competitive running and began drinking, only a little at first, then more and more. She certainly does not resemble an elite athlete today, but there is no way of telling what she looked like a decade ago. Now her face is pinched, her eyes sunken, and her body withered. Her arms are no bigger around than the bones within them, and her knees look uncommonly huge in the middle of her spindly legs.

She had told the admitting resident that she had received psychiatric care, but she refuses to give us details about her family and social background or other aspects of her life that might provide insight into her condition. Whatever her tragedies, she keeps them to herself, and no visitors have come in whom we might ask for information about her. She insists on being called Charlotte rather than Ms. Atkinson, which is unusual, and I wonder if she has entered the hospital using a phony name, believing that hospitalization reflects personal shame rather than ill health.

When she was first seen in the ICU three days ago, Charlotte's blood pressure was low from severe loss of blood; so she was given a large infusion of fluid through one of her veins and then a transfusion of two units of concentrated red blood cells. But because of the large volume of fluids that had to be administered intravenously to keep her blood pressure at a safe level, plus the markedly decreased amount of protein in her bloodstream due to her malnutrition, some of the fluid had overflowed from the blood vessels in her lungs into the tiny neighboring air sacs and swamped them, a common condition in the ICU called "pulmonary edema." This is a grave complication because it impairs breathing and the transfer of oxygen from the lungs into the bloodstream. The patient can drown in her own fluids. ICU doctors frequently cause or worsen pulmonary edema by giving too much blood, plasma, or other fluids intravenously.

Because of the pulmonary edema, we had to postpone an internal examination—an "endoscopy"—of the organs in her upper gastrointestinal tract. Endoscopy is done by passing a yard-long, snakelike fiberoptic instrument, an endoscope, through the mouth into the organs of the upper digestive tract, the esophagus, stomach, and duodenum, one after the other, and displaying the image of the interior of those organs on a television monitor. The procedure was carried out two days ago when Charlotte's lungs were less waterlogged, and it revealed eroded areas of black dead or dying tissue covering much of her esophagus. No source of bleeding was discovered. The ulceration was so severe and extensive that the endoscopist first thought that she must have swallowed lye or some other corrosive chemical. When the sedation wore off and she could talk, he asked her directly if she had taken anything. "No, no I didn't," she said in a soft but emphatic voice. "Nothing like that."

Everything seemed to settle down, and she had been transferred out of the unit. But suddenly, about two hours ago, blood began to erupt once again from her mouth, and back she came. When we arrive at her bedside, she is receiving her third unit of blood, and two more have been ordered. Fortunately, the repeat fiberoptic endoscopy is just starting. We all gather around the television screen to watch. Charlotte's charred and ulcerated esophagus is truly exceptional but does not appear to have changed from the day before yesterday. As before, we cannot see any site of active bleeding. This time, however, her stomach contains at least a quart of partially clotted blood. Because she is continuing to bleed, I am compelled to ask the surgeons to see Ms. Atkinson; so I tell the resident to call them. Sometimes an emergency operation is the only way to stop relentless hemorrhage.

Specialists in internal medicine interact with their colleagues in surgery all the time; we have a necessary and highly beneficial partnership. Each time we meet, though, internists tend to become a little edgy. Surgeons routinely perform technical feats no internist would ever conceive of undertaking, and they bring these brilliant skills with them when they consult on a patient. But they often bring their giant egos and short fuses as well. A surgeon friend of mine has characterized his confreres as "Often wrong, but never in doubt." By contrast, the call to arms for internists is "Don't just do something, stand there." It is undoubtedly good for the profession that it includes men and women of instant action as well as those of prolonged reflection; but when these polar temperaments meet at the bedside of a sick person, things can heat up.

Fortunately, the deliberations over Charlotte Atkinson did not result in a hot confrontation. Because no one had ever seen an esophagus like hers before, there was no personal experience—there was not even known precedent—to guide us; moreover, it was obvious from a glance at her bony face, shriveled breasts, and skeletal extremities—signs of malnutrition that were confirmed by the results of her laboratory tests—that she was a terrible candidate for the kind of extensive surgery that would be needed. Furthermore, we could not be absolutely certain that removal of much of her esophagus would cure her bleeding because we did not know exactly where the blood was coming from. Nothing causes more dissatisfaction and chagrin than subjecting a patient to a dangerous operation for ongoing hemorrhage only to have the bleeding continue afterward.

"Better hope she stops bleeding," the attending surgeon advised us. "We'll take her, but only if she bleeds briskly again and doesn't respond to more blood." In the back of my mind another thought emerged: was it possible that this victim of a self-destructive disorder was contributing to her own bleeding by taking anticoagulants or some other medication? I would review the results of her laboratory tests carefully with this in mind.

It is already 9:00 a.m. Thirty minutes each to review two newly admitted patients is not unusual, but today is the first of the month and every one of the seven patients in the unit is new to us. Leaving Charlotte to receive another transfusion, we go next to see Althanette Washington, a sixty-four-year-old unemployed woman, who is also suffering from a gastrointestinal hemorrhage and who is known from previous admissions to be a heavy drinker, with alcohol-induced scarring of the liver—alcoholic cirrhosis. She came to SFGH last night after vomiting material that resembled "coffee grounds" and passing stools that she described as "tarry," medical terminology she had evidently heard before, and both trademark signs of bleeding into the upper gastrointestinal tract. Fresh blood is recognizably red, but when blood remains long enough in the digestive system to become partially decomposed by juices in the stomach and intestine, it turns black. Mrs. Washington had lost enough blood to make her dizzy when she stood up, but when Dr. Quillici was questioning and examin-

ing her in the emergency department, he noticed her responses were a little off the mark and she kept drifting off to sleep. Bleeding into the gastrointestinal tract of someone with cirrhosis can cause torpor, but to make sure nothing else was amiss he ordered a computed tomographic (CT) x-ray study of her head, which was taken on her way to the ICU. Her "hematocrit," our routine measurement of the quantity of red blood cells circulating in the bloodstream, had plunged, so she was transfused a total of five units of blood last night.

By the time we see her, the gastroenterologists have already completed the fiberoptic endoscopic examination of Mrs. Washington's esophagus, stomach, and duodenum, and this demonstrated small esophageal "varices," which, as the name implies, are dilated lumpy veins similar to varicose veins in the leg. These varices form in the esophagus and stomach of patients with chronic advanced cirrhosis. They grow in an effort to reroute the blood flow that cannot get through the distorted veins in the scarred liver but often bleed torrentially. Later, when we review the CT films of her head in the x-ray department, we see that she also has a large abnormal lump in the middle part of her brain, a serious though probably benign tumor called a meningioma. We decide to keep her in the unit for another twenty-four hours to make sure the bleeding does not recur and to allow her to wake up more fully. The neurosurgeons, who have heard about her, are already circling, eager to attack her brain tumor. "We hear you've got a meningioma in here," says the chief resident in neurosurgery, leaning in at the door.

Next, we see the four patients who have been in the unit for several days or more. Two of them suffer from the same severe condition, long-standing lung disease of the asthma-bronchitis-emphysema type, which is also called chronic obstructive pulmonary disease. One of these patients has already been in the unit for over a month, the other for "only" a week. The long-timer, Truman Caughey, just thirty-five years old, is a former truck driver who had worked regularly until a year ago. Since then he has had many hospitalizations for res-

piratory failure, most of them severe enough to have required intubation. Several of his attacks seem to have been precipitated by sudden bouts of agitation that provoked wheezing and coughing. In the clinic and in the hospital, his physicians have carefully questioned him and his mother, with whom he lives and who helps take care of him, in hopes of unraveling the cause of these dramatic episodes. "Were you smoking at the time? Were cats or dogs in the room? Were there fumes or pollutants in the air?" But no trigger was ever found. Agitation can incite asthma and vice versa, and it is often problematic which comes first. Consider the intensity of the emotions that must be unleashed when you feel yourself slowly starting to smother, you realize it is probably going to get much worse, and you know you could die from it!

When we see him for the first time this morning, Mr. Caughey has been in the ICU for nearly five weeks and has required assisted ventilation almost the entire time. He has also needed intubation three times, because each time the tube is removed his asthma flares up again and he is unable to breathe by himself. Today, he is stuporous and does not wake up during our examination. I turn to his nurse, Imelda Tuazon, a dainty woman with a round, attractive face that appears fixed in a permanent smile. Although she sometimes sounds gruff ("Not now. Can't you see I'm busy?"), she has the proverbial heart of gold and will do anything for her patients and almost anything for the residents and students. Imelda, still smiling, explains, "This is because we have to give him large and frequent doses of fentanyl and midazolam (drugs used to relieve pain and anxiety). Every time the level of sedation drops, he goes wild and begins to wheeze and buck the ventilator. You'll see for yourself; it's dangerous. There's no alternative. We have to do it."

I meet his mother, an intelligent and concerned woman, who sits patiently by his bedside, hour after hour, though he is too sedated to know. She says, "It's obvious Truman's really sick. Please tell me the worst." When I tell her he might not make it through this hospitalization, she asks, "I smoked when he was a baby. Do you think I did it to him?" I point out that he has told his doctors that he is a heavy smoker, and that this is far more destructive to his lungs than her smoking many years ago. She tells me that she and her son have never

discussed the kind of care he has already received, much less the care he wants
in the future, even though he has been intubated and in ICUs many times. Like
many people, they find it impossible to face the issues of pain and death, even
when they are directly confronting them.

Truman Caughey has severe refractory asthma-bronchitis-emphysema,
but the reason he is in the ICU is because his lungs are unable to furnish
oxygen to and remove carbon dioxide from his body, a condition called
"respiratory failure." Normal breathing consists of the repeated inhala-
tion of fresh air and the uptake of oxygen into the lungs, followed by the
exhalation of stale air and the elimination of carbon dioxide. Besides the
lungs, respiration involves the brain, the muscles that inflate and deflate
the chest, and various sensors and connecting nerves, which collectively
constitute the respiratory system. Respiratory failure, a common condition in most ICUs, means that any of a multitude of abnormalities
within this tightly integrated system has led to inadequate uptake of oxygen, or to insufficient elimination of carbon dioxide, or, as Mr. Caughey
demonstrated, both.

I had no doubt that Mr. Caughey's respiratory failure was caused by
advanced, smoking-related, chronic obstructive pulmonary disease, but
it was also obvious that the problem was considerably aggravated by his
need for sedative and pain-killing drugs. These medications are among
the many two-edged swords in daily use in the ICU. Patients often
thrash around in their beds, struggle against the hated endotracheal tube
and ventilator, and may disconnect airway tubing or tear out cannulas
and catheters; heavy sedation quiets these dangerous movements and allows a breathing machine to work more efficiently. But heavy sedation
also depresses the brain and takes away the normal urge to breathe spontaneously, thereby causing an ICU catch-22 by prolonging the need for
intubation and machine-assisted breathing. In short, we will never be
able to "extubate" or remove the endotracheal tube from Mr. Caughey
and liberate him from the need for machine-assisted breathing so long

as he continues to receive such large doses of sedatives. Yet there is no way to get rid of these easily. Imelda, who knows what she is talking about, has warned me.

The other patient with asthma-bronchitis-emphysema is Howard McVicker, a sixty-three-year-old man who has been in the ICU one week. He also has refractory respiratory failure because of severe underlying chronic obstructive pulmonary disease, and he too requires heavy sedation to control his recurring bouts of thrashing, gasping, and evident panic. To make matters worse, when he is restless his blood pressure climbs to alarming levels and his heart rate not only accelerates but at times becomes irregular. Jack Cramer, Mr. McVicker's nurse, who knows him well, says, "Howard's doing fine, and now's the time to lighten his sedation a little"; this is welcome news that will allow us to push forward with vigorous efforts to get him to breathe on his own. We set up a plan with Jack and the respiratory therapist to cut back the sedatives and, as Mr. McVicker gradually wakes up, to reduce the amount of support provided by the machine to the level of independence he is able to tolerate.

Next, another resident fills me in about Patrick Guzman, a forty-year-old house painter with a long history of chronic alcoholism complicated by cirrhosis. Because of his steady heavy drinking, his liver disease has been relentlessly progressive. Last week he had a brief admission to the ICU for a brisk gastrointestinal hemorrhage. This time he is dying.

Patients with advanced cirrhosis are exceptionally fragile: they are susceptible to a host of complications, of which hemorrhage and infection are among the most common and dangerous. When either of these occurs, it often causes a backlash reaction in the liver that worsens its already compromised function. This happened to Mr. Guzman shortly after he arrived. His jaundice in-

creased, his blood failed to clot, and he developed marked swelling of his belly and legs from retained fluid. Four days ago, he became confused and then comatose; next, his lungs began to accumulate fluid, now frank pulmonary edema, for which an endotracheal tube had to be inserted so his breathing could be assisted with a ventilator. Last night, his kidneys virtually stopped making urine.

Today, he shows florid evidence of marked liver failure, and his blood pressure is beginning to decrease. It is clear he is close to death. We give this terrible news to his two brothers, who are by his bedside. They tell us, with disarming composure, "Pat always said he never wanted to be kept alive on machines." We all agree that he should be allowed to die as comfortably as possible, which means without the endotracheal tube and ventilator.

To let Patrick Guzman die quietly is an easy decision for two reasons. Above all, there is no hope for the recovery of his destroyed liver, an indispensable organ that regulates metabolism, destroys toxins, and produces vital circulating substances. He is not a candidate for liver transplantation because he continued to drink up to the day of his hospitalization. Some transplant centers will accept steady drinkers; others, like ours, require at least six months' abstinence, and even then it is debatable if alcoholics have a prognosis that justifies this elaborate and costly procedure. Because further medical care is futile, we can legally discontinue his treatment. The judgment that additional aggressive treatment would be futile is not always so easy to make, but there is no doubt here. Not only has Mr. Guzman not responded to vigorous therapy; he has deteriorated markedly despite his being treated with all we have to offer.

The second reason for our easy decision is provided by his brothers' telling us that Mr. Guzman has clearly stated he does not want machine-assisted breathing and that the family wants it stopped. Although verbal declarations of this sort are not binding, we are glad to hear them because they eliminate the threat of confrontation when physicians conclude that a situation is futile yet the family expects a miracle.

Around noon, after his brothers' wives and a few cousins have arrived, the endotracheal tube is removed from his windpipe, and a morphine infusion is started to make him more comfortable. Morphine also helps by preventing the reflex gasps and agonal muscle contractions that signal fast-approaching death, which the family may interpret as hideous suffering. Relief of unendurable pain and torment is one of medicine's oldest and strongest imperatives, and morphine is ideal for this purpose; it comforts the patient directly and the family indirectly.

After the family has gathered at the bedside, Molly Wolford, the head nurse, goes in and turns off the television screen that displays Mr. Guzman's blood pressure, heart rate, and electrocardiographic tracing. "Why are you doing that?" one of his brothers asks.

"We don't need this information any longer," she replies; "we do better without it." But Molly does not disconnect the monitor at the central nurses' station because we must know what is going on at all times. She turns the bedside monitor off because we have learned that relatives and friends tend to pay more attention to it than to their loved one. People become obsessed watching the electrocardiographic squiggles that announce each heartbeat marching across the screen. Although the physiological nuances are undoubtedly overlooked, the deeper meaning of the electrical signals of life is hard to miss when they slow in frequency, gradually widen in appearance, and then finally stop altogether.

The last person for us to see, Constancia Noe, is barely nineteen years old and in some ways the most difficult of our seven patients. She is a small woman who has a tube in her windpipe for machine-assisted breathing; a tube in the right side of her chest to keep the lung on that side expanded; a tube that goes through her nose and stomach into her intestine for feeding; a tube in her bladder to drain and measure urine; a tube in an artery in her right wrist to measure her blood pressure and sample blood; and two tubes in forearm veins for administering fluids and medications. Even though she has lost a lot of weight and is aged in appearance, it is easy to imagine that she was once very pretty, with an almond face, dark eyes, and long black hair. Now she is barely responsive: she too has received a lot of sedation.

Despite her youth, Mrs. Noe has a long history of serious complications related to excess alcohol and heavy use of intravenous heroin, cocaine, and other uppers and downers—medical conditions ranging from pancreatitis and episodes of bleeding from her stomach to fractured bones from falling. Then, nine months before this hospitalization, she developed Pneumocystis carinii *pneumonia and was diagnosed with AIDS. Now, she has features of advanced HIV disease, despite her having been treated with all the available anti-HIV medications, none of which she has ever taken regularly.*

Although the cause of her pneumonia was promptly identified and treated, she has done poorly. When she came to us for breathing support, her right lung had collapsed from an internal rupture of a small cyst that allowed air to escape from the lung and accumulate around it. To re-expand the lung, we had to insert a large-bore tube through her rib cage into the chest cavity and connect it to a suction machine and drainage apparatus that hangs at her bedside.

I have no choice but to continue the treatment started by her other physicians. I would like to talk to her family about her dismal prognosis, but I cannot speak frankly. To the doctors who talked to her at the beginning of this hospitalization, she made her views unmistakably clear: "I've got AIDS for a long time, but my family don't know about it, and I don't want them to know about it now." I am quite sure she is going to die, but if she instructed us to be aggressive, we might prolong her life a few weeks and get her back on treatment. At this point, though, we cannot find out what she wants because she is too sick and sedated to tell us.

Ward rounds and x-ray rounds finally finish a little after 11:30 A.M., but the day is far from over. I will make a note in the chart of every patient, which today will probably take several hours because I have to read completely through each current record. When I make my notes, I commandeer one of the barstool-like chairs that stands just outside each of the rooms; these lofty seats allow the nurses to watch their charges through a window while entering data into a nearby computer that stores the daily reports. On this perch I have easy access to the computer for the information I need to write my notes in the patient's medical record, but I also make an easy target for anyone who wants to ask a question, get advice, or just chat. And people do, all the time.

The position outside the patient's room also means that family and friends inside can see me, so I always go in to have a few words with whoever is there. Because all this takes extra time, I am unable to finish my notes until nearly 3:00 P.M., when I buy a sandwich in the hospital's coffee shop. I slip into my office to eat it, while returning phone calls and dealing with essentials: a typical ICU day.

About 4:00 P.M. I go back to the units to check up on things. The respiratory therapist says, "I've made good progress in weaning Jisoo Hong from the ventilator," so I tell him to take her endotracheal tube out.

Smiling Imelda Tuazon indicates that Charlotte Atkinson is receiving her fourth unit of blood, and "She hasn't turned a hair."

I notice that Patrick Guzman's breathing is typically agonal, with slow and shallow gasps. I speak with one of his brothers, who has come out to see me. "I think it will be over soon. How are you holding up?"

"The sooner the better," he mutters. "This is much harder than I thought it would be. But, listen—and my brother joins me in this— everyone here has been terrific. It makes things much easier."

"Be sure to tell that to the nurses," I reply, "they are the ones to thank." People rarely thank us for a death.

At 6:30 P.M., before leaving, I go back and see everyone again, this time with Ella Andrews, and I am gladdened by her voluble enthusiasm. Mrs. Hong is breathing well by herself, having been extubated. Mr. Guzman is dead, and his family has gone. I meet one of Constancia Noe's brothers and talk a little with him, though I am careful not to mention AIDS. Everything else is quiet and there are no new patients. I take off.

I arrive home thirteen hours after I left for the hospital this morning.

I start to miss my wife as I walk into our house. She went to France on business two days ago and will be gone all month. I feed our cat Walter and open a beer. It has been a long day, and I am on call tonight and for the rest of the month; I will wear my beeper everywhere I go. But at least I am home and not in the hospital, like Ella and the others, who not only have to be there but will probably be up most of the time. I'll go back to the ICU if they need me, but that doesn't happen often at night.

The key people in any ICU are the nurses, like Molly Wolford, Imelda Tuazon, and Jack Cramer. These motivated and proficient women and men are specially trained for their demanding responsibilities in an eight-week course that mixes classroom teaching and supervised preceptorship in the units. Trainees emerge from the indoctrination as "novice" ICU nurses, which means they can work in an ICU but require extra support and guidance. After two years of apprenticeship, their experience qualifies them to work in any unit completely on their own.

One nurse generally takes care of two patients, never more. When a patient requires even greater vigilance, the ratio is one to one. During emergencies or complicated procedures, two or more nurses may attend a single patient. According to this formula, the number of nurses in the ICU on a given day depends on how many patients are there and how sick they are. Around-the-clock coverage is facilitated by having the nurses work twelve-hour shifts, either daytime or nighttime, instead of the usual nursing pattern of three shifts of eight hours each. ICU nurses are paid more than other nurses, and they earn the difference. They provide most of the care—monitoring temperature and blood pressure, giving medications, weighing and bathing patients, recording the innumerable clinical details—and they are the main communicators with patients and their families. Nurses also have a lot of responsibility for making independent decisions and acting on them—for example, when a patient's heart stops or beats chaotically.

Our essential full-time staff also includes a respiratory therapist, another specially trained professional who sets up and regulates the breathing machines. At any one time, one third to one half the patients in our ICU are being mechanically ventilated, and at one time or another almost all patients are given extra oxygen to breathe; so respiratory therapists, like nurses, play indispensable roles and have considerable independent responsibility.

Today should be a little more relaxed than yesterday because there has been only one new admission, and because two of yesterday's patients are gone (Patrick Guzman died and Jisoo Hong was transferred). The new medical residents and students will have a chance to get acquainted with the nurses and respiratory therapists with whom they will work the rest of the month, and from whom they have much to learn.

Ella Andrews, bubbling despite an active night on call, herds us to Gyula Vysinsky's room and introduces me to the first-year resident who admitted her. He tells us her story. "Gyula is a seventy-six-year-old immigrant from Hungary, who probably had a convulsion; after she collapsed on a sidewalk in downtown San Francisco, someone called 911. But when the ambulance arrived, no one was there to explain what had happened." So we don't know for sure.

After intubating her, the admitting staff contacted her husband and learned the name of her private physician. Ella called him and found out that Mrs. Vysinsky, a heavy cigarette smoker, has been under his care for many years for pulmonary emphysema and chronic bronchitis. Her condition had been stable until about six weeks ago when she visited his office complaining of worsening chronic cough that produced more phlegm than usual. After a chest x-ray showed a lump in her right lung, plans were made to evaluate her for cancer of the lung, but she did not show up for her appointments.

Mrs. Vysinsky is a plump, hale-looking woman with shining white hair combed over a bald spot, like a man. She is beginning to wake up, but she is restless and keeps pulling at the restraints on her hands and feet, put there to keep her from pulling out the breathing tube or falling out of bed. Her chest x-ray shows a golf-ball-size mass in the upper portion of her right lung, highly suggestive of a malignancy. Worse, her head CT scan reveals several defects in her brain that are almost certainly metastases, malignant deposits from the spread of a primary cancer of the lung. Our plan is to allow her to awaken further and, as soon as she can breathe by herself, to remove the endotracheal tube. Then, once she is stable, we will send her to the private hospital where her personal physician has already asked to have her transferred. She will be no worse for her brief brush with our unit, but she has a dim future ahead of her.

For decades, lung cancer has been the most common cause of death from malignancy among men in the United States; since 1987, it has surpassed breast cancer as the most common cause of death from malignancy among women as well. Impressive new data indicate that women are even more susceptible than men to the cancer-producing effects of cigarette smoke;[1] this means that lung cancer may appear in women at a lower level of smoking than in men and often at an earlier age. As nearly everyone knows, the majority of cancers of the lung (at least eighty-five percent) are caused by tobacco smoke, and thus the disease could largely be prevented if people would only stop smoking or, better yet, never smoke at all.

The finding by Mrs. Vysinsky's personal physician of a new abnormality on the chest x-ray taken six weeks ago reinforces the old clinical admonition that I repeated for the housestaff during rounds: always consider the possibility of lung cancer in a habitual smoker whose chronic cough worsens. Because of Mrs. Vysinsky's recalcitrance in keeping her appointments, the diagnosis has not yet been proven by obtaining a specimen of tissue and examining it under the microscope. Such resistance to diagnosis happens all the time: people behave as though deep down they know what is wrong with them but are terrified of having the unpleasant truth revealed. Nevertheless, we are convinced that she has lung cancer that has spread to her brain, one of the most common and devastating sites of metastases. A brain metastasis is also the best explanation for her putative convulsion. It all fits. Unfortunately, as Mrs. Vysinsky demonstrates, by the time symptoms develop in most of lung cancer's victims, the malignancy is already so widespread that it is no longer curable. We cannot discuss this with her because she is not awake enough to understand; her own doctor will have the grim duty of breaking the dreadful news.

As we decided yesterday after consultation with the gastroenterologists and surgeons, Charlotte Atkinson, the young woman with bulimia, has been treated with conservative medical measures: drugs to block acid secretion by the stomach, feedings through a tube positioned just beyond the stomach in the duodenum to bypass her damaged esophagus, and more blood. The results of her laboratory tests show nothing to suggest she has deliberately taken medications to prevent her blood from clotting, as I had mistrustfully considered. In fact, today she has stopped bleeding and has done so well that we think it safe to move her back to a regular ward for further medical and psychiatric care. I tell her, "There's a good chance you'll get well and stay well, but you have to quit drinking and cooperate with the psychiatrists."

She smiles and says in a tottery voice, "I already know that."

Ms. Atkinson had severe esophagitis, but its exact cause was never determined. The best explanation for her disorder is bulimia with its well-known cycle of eating followed by protracted self-induced vomiting; sometimes little or no food is ingested but vomiting is initiated anyway. The act of vomiting causes reflux into the esophagus of hydrochloric acid, a powerful corrosive chemical that is normally secreted by the stomach to aid in digestion. Looking back now, the decision not to subject her to what would have been a risky operation was wise. She remained in the hospital three weeks, including a week of intensive psychiatric therapy. The day before she was discharged, a third fiberoptic examination of her esophagus showed marked improvement. Her medical future remains uncertain, however, largely because of the bulimia.

Internists are good at treating the medical complications of bulimia, but not the condition itself. Our ignorance about this strange sickness is frustrating, and even psychiatrists have difficulty unraveling the complex interacting conditions that lie behind bulimia, including depression, a high need for control, addiction to perfection, self-esteem problems, and rage at authority. Although Ms. Atkinson had already failed several attempts at inpatient and outpatient psychiatric treatment for her disorder, now at least she has another chance to benefit from the comprehensive services offered at SFGH.

Truman Caughey, our refractory asthmatic who has been in the unit for five weeks, has had a fairly good day. I suggest minor adjustments to his breathing machine in an effort to coax him to breathe more on his own. I give his mother, continuously at his bedside, the report of minimal improvement. "Just keep trying, Doc," she implores. "Please save him. He's all I've got." To myself I say, I hope that's not true because I'm not sure I can save him. Pure asthma is eminently treatable, but when combined with chronic obstructive pulmonary disease as severe as his, it's problematic.

Our other patient with serious asthma-bronchitis-emphysema, Howard Mc-Vicker, has also had a quiet twenty-four hours. We think we have made a good start in weaning him from the ventilator, so we change the settings on his ma-chine to force him to breathe a little bit more by himself. Jim Shotinger, who has the duty today and tonight, seizes Mr. McVicker's chart to write the order for the respiratory therapist. I notice that Jim is left-handed, as am I, but he cocks his left wrist high in the air in an awkward fashion, much different from the way I write, thanks to a strict first-grade teacher who used a ruler to whack my wrist if it strayed.

Our young patient with multiple complications of advanced AIDS, Constancia Noe, is more awake and alert this morning, though not able to communicate because of the tube in her windpipe and the need for sedation. We are sending more specimens of secretions to the laboratory in hopes of identifying the cause of what appears to be a worsening pneumonia. We are also stopping the suction on her chest tube to find out if her right lung will remain expanded by itself, as it must before the tube can be removed.

Yesterday afternoon, I met with the chairman of our hospital's Ethics Com-mittee, Dr. Richard Broderick, to discuss my concerns about her. We desperately want guidance in determining what we should do if, as seems inevitable, her condition deteriorates. Should we insert more chest tubes if her other lung col-lapses? Should we use medications to support her blood pressure if it drops? Should we pound on her chest and shock her heart if it stops beating? These are all real prospects. I can't stop thinking about how she's only nineteen years old. Would even a few more weeks of life mean something to her?

"We have another tough one," I told him. "A young woman with AIDS who is steadily losing ground and will probably die soon. We need to decide how ag-gressive to be. But she's in no shape to tell us, and she told everyone at the be-ginning of this hospitalization not to discuss matters with her family because she doesn't want them to know she has AIDS. There was and perhaps still is a Mr. Noe, but he abandoned her and vanished a few months after their mar-riage. I'd like to talk to her father to try to find out if he has any indication

about how she wants to be treated. But she has clearly said not to. What do we do now?"

Today, Dr. Broderick comes to the ICU to tell us that he has thought about our predicament and talked to others on his committee. Their conclusion is that, despite her explicit interdiction, we can disclose the fact that she has AIDS to her father. To serve as her surrogate and advise us medically on her behalf, he must be informed of the exact situation.

I see the logic, but I am uneasy with this decision because of its contradiction of Mrs. Noe's stated wishes. Yet we do not have much time. I turn to her nurse, Pauline Victoria, who knows the family well and who has excellent rapport with them. I ask her please to call Constancia's father and make an appointment for me to meet with him and any of her brothers and sisters who want to join us.

She fixes her deep blue eyes on me with their most piercing gaze and nods OK. Pauline has worked in the ICU for several years and is a superior nurse, but something about her has changed. Her gogglelike stare has become so intense lately that I worry that her thyroid gland may be overactive.

Ethics Committees operate in more than sixty percent of United States hospitals with at least two hundred beds. Their chief functions are to educate clinical staff and patients about ethical matters in medicine, to assist in developing institutional policies, and to consult on ethical problems in patient care. The legal weight of counsel from ethics committees, however, is unclear. Especially murky is the question whether their advice should shield physicians who follow it from civil and criminal liability.[2]

Our Ethics Committee at SFGH, in place since 1987, has always provided me with good advice, ranging from defining legal responsibilities as a physician to suggesting psychological techniques with families. The committee is careful not to say exactly what to do, but it does define the ethical and legal boundaries in which to operate. In the case of Constancia Noe, the group's guidance is valuable and educational. Most medical ethicists believe that patient autonomy is a key principle. According to

Dr. Richard Broderick, though, honoring her autonomy in this situation creates operational conflicts: we want to follow her instructions not to inform her family; yet we need her guidance, and her father might know her wishes. Even if he does not, he cannot serve as her surrogate in these grim circumstances without knowing precisely what the circumstances are.

Much later, when my wife, with whom I sometimes discuss matters of this sort, learned of the Ethics Committee's recommendation to tell Mrs. Noe's father, she was shocked. "What's the point of encouraging patients to let you know what they want done if you ignore their wishes?" she objected. "If that woman had been a man, would you have overruled his directives?" She doubted it. "And all this so her father could decide, thereby infantilizing her and denying her the autonomy you doctors are so concerned about. It might as well be the nineteenth century," she sniffed. This has prompted me to reconsider the issues. At the time of writing this, I think I erred in telling her father.

Althanette Washington, our patient with gastrointestinal hemorrhage and a previously unsuspected brain tumor, has awakened nicely, her blood pressure has remained stable, and she appears to have stopped bleeding. "How are you today, Mrs. Washington?" I ask.

"Doin' good," she replies. She is pleased when I tell her that everything is going well and that we plan to transfer her to a medical ward later this morning. When I remind her about the tumor and the need for a big operation, she says, "I'll think about it."

The first intensive care unit anywhere was organized in the summer of 1952, a few months after I finished medical school, at the beginning of the last worldwide epidemic of poliomyelitis. This was the worst outbreak of polio in history, judged from the number of persons stricken, both children and adults, and from the extent of their paralysis. There was an urgent need to provide breathing assistance to the hundreds of patients whose respiratory muscles had been paralyzed by the disease or whose brains were affected, but there was a shortage of breathing machines, and those that were available, chiefly iron lungs, were cumbersome and inefficient.

To cope with the worsening problem in Denmark, a special unit was organized in Copenhagen to introduce new techniques of helping polio victims breathe. Rubber tubes were inserted through surgically made holes in the neck and sealed in the patients' windpipes, so that oxygen-enriched air could be forced into their lungs by repeatedly squeezing— by hand—an elastic bag, twenty-four hours a day. At first, teams of local medical students, working four shifts of six hours each, took turns doing the squeezing, as long as it was needed, usually a few months for each patient. At one time, seventy polio patients in the Copenhagen hospital required manual breathing assistance.[3] Danish physiologists quickly improved on the complicated research methods for measuring the carbon dioxide and acid-base status of blood and established the first clinical system for monitoring the effectiveness of assisted breathing. Once these techniques were in place, the mortality rate plummeted from ninety percent to twenty-five percent. Given this impressive result, the value of a new type of breathing machine, one that would push air into the lungs, as the medical students were doing with their hands, was recognized, and a prototype ventilator was developed with incredible speed and in use by 1953.

Since then, the goal of intensive care—to provide high-quality medical and nursing care for critically ill patients—has not changed, nor has the team approach, though the equipment and facilities have improved substantially. In most moderate-size community hospitals there is a single ICU for both medical and surgical patients, but in larger and more active hospitals the two units are often physically and administratively separate. A derivative of a medical ICU is a coronary care unit, in which medical patients with acute or severe heart disease are cared for. Depending on local institutional practices and demands, intensive care units can be operated exclusively for newborn babies, pediatric patients, neurosurgical patients, patients after heart surgery, burn patients, or any other specially designated group.

DAY	
3	*Saturday*

Saturday already. Life goes on as usual in the ICU so far as the patients are concerned, but today there are a few changes: the two head nurses take the weekend off; daily assignments of the residents are varied so that some can have a well-earned day of rest on either Saturday or Sunday; and only two of our three third-year residents make ward rounds with me. Today, it is Ian Trent-Johnson's turn to be on call, his first of the month. Bespectacled, with a serious demeanor and abundant black hair always in need of a trim, he looks like the Cambridge-educated scholar he is reputed to be. But, unlike his American counterparts, he is quiet and contemplative. Ian seldom speaks up, but when he does all his fellow residents pay close attention. The weekend schedule means that after we finish rounds this morning Jim Shotinger can leave the hospital and take the entire weekend off. Robust but slightly klutzy, Jim greatly prefers sports to sleep, and, like many of the residents, he is crazy about wind-surfing. He plans to spend several hours today and tomorrow pounding the waves of San Francisco Bay, where there is always a reliable breeze, though his lack of coordination worries me. It is not unusual for medical students and housestaff, surrounded by so much ill health, to indulge rather obsessively in physical activity. They kayak in the summer, ski in the winter, and jog all year long. Travel is popular, especially to the Napa Valley wine country north of the city for picnics. Although chronically sleep-deprived, residents spend surprisingly little time resting. Hardly anyone studies.

Many of the attending faculty, including me, play tennis as a way of staying in shape and deactivating. I have a game lined up late this afternoon and another one tomorrow.

■

As soon as I walk through the door of the unit, Jim Shotinger, who is conspicuously anxious to leave, picks up the phone and pages the team that has admitted the two new patients. The first of these is Hanako Furukawa, a ninety-five-year-old Japanese mother of four. She was brought by ambulance from a nursing home after she had been found completely unresponsive in her bed. According to the night supervisor who discovered her, Mrs. Furukawa was ordinarily lively and communicative and, despite having to use a walker because of arthritis, was constantly shuffling from room to room to chat with her cronies. In the emergency ward she was deeply comatose and in respiratory failure. Jim Shotinger immediately called the first of her children on the next-of-kin list, her eldest son, to ask how aggressive her care should be. "We want everything done, of course," the son said anxiously. After Jim explained about the painful tube, the son cried, "Yes, yes. Go ahead. Do it! I'll get my brother and sisters and we'll be right over."

When we see Mrs. Furukawa, she is intubated and being ventilated. She is a tiny, thin woman with a twisted spine and lopsided chest. When I listen to her lungs they sound full of gurgling secretions. When I press hard on her breastbone or pinch her skin, she contracts the muscles of her arms and legs in a characteristic extension posture—a primitive reflex, without purpose or sentience, and a classic sign of severe damage to vital parts of the brain. Her chest x-ray shows a tortuous spine ("scoliosis") and probable pneumonia.

The CT (computed tomographic) examination of her head is normal, so there is no obvious explanation for her coma. She also appears to have pneumo-

nia, probably from aspiration of saliva and other regurgitated material from her stomach into her lungs. We have no choice but to continue to treat and support her—her son insists on an aggressive approach. While waiting to see what happens, we will push to liberate her from the ventilator and get the tube out of her windpipe as soon as she can breathe on her own. I will talk with her entire family, to impress on them the direness of the situation and the likelihood of a worsening course.

Nearly everyone knows that the proportion of people who live to be sixty-five years of age or older is steadily increasing in the United States and many other industrialized countries. Moreover, although the elderly constitute thirteen percent of our population, they account for thirty-three percent of all expenditures for health care, much of it spent during the last year of life. Some question whether a person ninety-five years old should be treated in an ICU, but most ICU experts agree that old age per se should not deny anyone admission. The severity and types of a patient's diseases are much better predictors of successful treatment in an ICU than is age alone.

By the severity measure, Hanako Furukawa, with deep coma complicated by pneumonia and respiratory failure, sufficient to require intubation and ventilation, does not seem to belong in our ICU. Yet her son wants "everything done," and so far it has been. Perhaps he is illustrating the phenomenon that families are apt to be more zealous in seeking aggressive care than are the elderly patients for whom they are supposedly speaking, but there is no way of knowing.

Our second new patient, Hugh Martini, is a thirty-three-year-old stage designer from San Francisco who had been complaining of rapidly progressive shortness of breath and an irritating dry cough. "Hugh decided to come to SFGH when he noticed his fingers were blue, and the ER docs picked up on him quickly, because he was unusually engaging and perceptive, even ani-

mated. But," adds the resident, "his ability to speak was compromised by the need to gasp for breath every few seconds." In the emergency department his hands, toes, ears, and lips were indeed a dusky bluish color, and the reason why was quickly established when the doctors found an extremely low level of oxygen in his arterial blood. He was in severe respiratory failure. Fortunately, the respiratory therapist contrived a special face mask and oxygen-delivery system, so it was not necessary to intubate him. His chest x-ray shows extensive abnormalities in both lungs that are strongly suggestive of Pneumocystis carinii, *still one of the most common ways for AIDS to declare itself. Jim Shotinger has wisely started him on the antibiotics-of-choice for pneumocystis pneumonia, and, because of Mr. Martini's severe respiratory failure, Jim has also given him prednisone, a cortisonelike drug that attenuates its severity.*

The resident from the team that admitted Mr. Martini and will follow him through his hospitalization has already reported to me that she has ascertained that he is gay and that he has not been tested for HIV infection, the underlying cause of AIDS. Asking patients direct questions about once supersensitive matters, such as sexual orientation and practices and whether they have ever had a sexually transmitted disease or been tested for HIV infection, is now routine when obtaining a medical history. The answers are crucial and greatly influence the initial diagnostic formulation and treatment. I have a feeling there is more in Mr. Martini's history than he is owning up to, so I try an indirect approach by asking him if he has ever had shingles, thrush, or pneumonia, well-established premonitory AIDS diseases. To each question, between gulps of oxygen, he replies no.

Hugh Martini is a sexually active gay man, and we are assuming he is infected with HIV. But we are not certain of this diagnosis or of the presence of *P. carinii* pneumonia, because several other AIDS-related conditions could cause identical abnormalities. He agrees to have the HIV blood test performed, but the results will not be available for several days. Knowing if one is HIV-positive has major therapeutic ramifications. I wonder why he has never been tested; he is clearly intelligent.

Most gay men in San Francisco are well informed about what constitutes high-risk sex, the natural history of HIV infection and AIDS, and available treatments, both approved and alternative. Perhaps Mr. Martini is like Gyula Vysinsky, just down the hall, in that he senses what is wrong but can't face knowing the truth.

Whatever the explanation, our immediate problem is to confirm the tentative diagnosis of pneumocystis pneumonia by studying secretions from his lungs and identifying the causative parasites. As so often happens when it is important to know right now, this is Saturday and the examination cannot be performed until Monday when the Microbiology-Parasitology Laboratory is open and the experts are available. While waiting over the weekend to find out what he has, we hope that his fragile ability to oxygenate will not worsen. If it does, he will require intubation, an intervention that will clearly indicate that his disease has progressed from severe but manageable to more likely fatal. In the grim figures of available statistics, his chance of surviving this episode of pneumonia will have decreased by more than half.

Truman Caughey, one of our two long-term patients with asthma-bronchitis-emphysema, has not changed much. Imelda Tuazon confirms, "We aren't getting anywhere in decreasing Truman's sedation. Every time I cut back, he bucks around like a bronco and begins to wheeze. Then the ventilator starts popping off, and I have to snow him again."

Our other patient with asthma complicating chronic obstructive pulmonary disease, Howard McVicker, did well most of yesterday with only minimal assistance from his breathing machine. When we examine him today, he is awake and alert and nods his head in response to questions. He also takes big breaths and will try to cough when I ask him to; his lungs sound improved and his chest x-ray has remained stable. He is ready for extubation. Beforehand, he will be given another vigorous aerosol treatment with antiasthma ("bronchodilator") medications, and his air passages will be suctioned free of secretions by passing a small plastic catheter through the endotracheal tube, first into one lung and then the other, to clean them thoroughly. Then, the respiratory therapist will take the tube out. If he does well, we will talk with him and his wife tonight, when she visits, about whether we should put the tube back, should he need it again.

Extubating a patient like Mr. McVicker is more an act of faith than of science. There are certain rules to follow, but they are far from absolute. I have had patients who, after flunking every test we tried as a guide to extubation, in desperation yanked the tube out themselves. (This is not a recommended maneuver because the balloon at the end of the tube remains inflated, and when pulled through the vocal cords the knob of latex can damage them.) Afterward, many of these patients breathed well by themselves and did not require reintubation. By contrast, other patients who were by all criteria ready for extubation were unable to breathe more than a few hours on their own after the tube was removed, and it had to be replaced. Most of the time things are straightforward, but sometimes it is remarkably difficult to judge what will happen.

Because Mr. McVicker has been intubated a long time (ten days), we have proceeded slowly and cautiously to see if he is truly ready for extubation. But as I explained to the residents during ward rounds, I had no doubt that the outcome depended more on the unpredictable nature of his volatile agitation-provoked wheezing and accompanying respiratory failure than on the exact moment we took the tube out.

Our desperately ill patient with AIDS, Constancia Noe, is steadily worsening. When I examine her, I can feel tiny bubbles of air in her neck and upper chest

*squishing around under my fingertips; this means that her right lung has col-
lapsed again and air has leaked from within the right chest cavity into the
neighboring tissues. She has obviously not tolerated our turning off the suction
connected to her chest tube, but when we turn it back on, a large continuous flow
of air that had not been present before comes through the tube. Either the original rupture in her lung has reopened or another one has occurred. This complication makes an already bad situation much worse because it means she
has failed to respond to all of our therapeutic efforts. I am sure she is dying,
and her family must be told. When they come this afternoon for the scheduled
meeting, I will inform them and will include the information about her having AIDS, so that they can tell us, if they know, how Mrs. Noe would want
us to proceed: to fight on or give up. Fortunately, Pauline Victoria, who has
cared for Mrs. Noe on several occasions and who knows her and her family better than others on staff, is on duty today and will lend a hand when we break
the news.*

The appointment time comes and goes with no sign of Mr. Palacio,
Constancia Noe's father, and the other members of her family. This is
unexpected because they have been attentive and faithful during her
long stay in the ICU. When they finally arrive more than an hour late,
trembling and visibly distressed, we learn that they have been delayed by
an accident a few blocks from the hospital. Their car was hit from behind by another car, and during the unpleasant scene that followed,
Mr. Palacio was threatened with a gun by the drunk driver of the other
car. The police arrived soon afterward and arrested the miscreant, but
the questions and reports took a long time, and all of the family are still
shaky. It is a terrible time to tell them that Mrs. Noe has AIDS and will
soon be dead. Full of remorse, I break the news. No one expresses shock
or surprise. Her father says, "Yeah, we know that. She's had it a long
time. But she didn't want us to know, so we didn't talk about it." Pauline,
who has spent many anxious moments with the family, deliberately
avoiding the subject of AIDS, is stunned; I can tell because she stops
staring at Mr. Palacio and lowers her gaze.

Gyula Vysinsky, whose presumed lung cancer has metastasized to her brain, perked up enough to be successfully extubated yesterday morning after rounds. She is still in the ICU because for several hours her heartbeat was irregular and rapid; fortunately, her blood pressure remained stable and did not decrease during the episode, as can happen. She remains confused and mumbles in Hungarian. Nothing else is changed. Her husband, a small dark man with huge bushy eyebrows, who was with her all day yesterday and is here again this morning, keeps saying, "I told her to stop smoking; I told her over and over."

Three hundred eighty-nine years ago, King James I of England condemned smoking as a "custome lothsome to the eye, hatefull to the Nose, harmefull to the braine, dangerous to the Lungs," and compared it to "the horrible Stigian smoke of the pit that is bottomlesse." He was right.

DAY	
4	*Sunday*

Great cities have great city hospitals. San Francisco is no exception. The present SFGH is a direct descendant of the first, supposedly temporary, infirmary established in 1850 during a cholera epidemic. In 1872, a new city hospital was dedicated at its present location south of Market Street. Patients with bubonic plague were treated here, first in 1900 and again in 1908. After the hospital became infested with rats and plague-carrying fleas, the buildings were burned and the patients were moved to a temporary facility located in an old racetrack. The replacement hospital was built in 1911, and the new medical center with its ICUs was inaugurated in 1976.

As the physical facilities improved, the hospital's mission gradually expanded from pesthouse to a place where comprehensive care is provided for the poor and the mentally ill, a role it still fulfills. Beginning in the 1950s, SFGH started to gain renown for its emergency department and battle-ready trauma service, which are now world-famous and among the busiest in California. Anyone who happens to be in San Francisco when injury or illness strikes can receive care at SFGH. We have a Regional Poison Control Center that provides information and advice each year to more than seventy thousand callers from ten counties in Northern California; the head of the Poison Center and his staff are also immensely helpful to us when patients with drug toxicity or drug overdosage are in the ICU. When it was recognized that San Francisco was one of the epicenters of the emerging AIDS epidemic, the city and its hospital reacted quickly by opening in 1983 the first AIDS outpatient clinic and, six months later, the first AIDS ward in the country. Our AIDS program rapidly became a national model for treatment, research, and community involvement. For eight straight years, SFGH was recognized by the editors of *US News & World Report* as one of the top medical centers in the United States, and the best of all for AIDS. This explains why Constancia Noe and Hugh Martini have been treated in our ICU. Another patient with AIDS is here this morning, and I am sure there will be many more.[1]

One of our new patients is Rosalie Larragasada, a forty-eight-year-old homeless woman, who is known to be a heavy drinker and heroin user and who hangs out in bars and addicts' "shooting galleries" in the nearby Mission district. Her anxious first-year resident reports that she has had many visits to SFGH for cirrhosis, skin infections, and gastrointestinal bleeding. Just two weeks ago, a large abscess in her thigh was drained by surgeons in the clinic. The resident explains, "Rosalie showed up late yesterday afternoon after vomiting coffee grounds. She came directly to us after the ER noticed that she was jaundiced and confused and that she had a swollen abdomen and chronic infection of the skin on her legs.

"After she got up here, I tapped her belly and got junky-looking fluid that was full of pus, but the lab couldn't find bugs [bacteria]. We started her on the usual cocktail [of antibiotics] for SBP [shorthand for "spontaneous bacterial peritonitis," a well-known and serious infectious complication of cirrhosis]. Her numbers [the results of laboratory tests] show horrible function of her liver, but heme-wise [blood count] her crit [hematocrit] hasn't dwindled but is an amazing thirty-four [high for someone in her condition, as normal for a woman is thirty-five to forty-five percent]."

By the time we see Ms. Larragasada, it is evident that her bleeding is not nearly as severe as originally feared, and her other problems have stabilized. The resident wants to keep her in the ICU at least another day because she is "so sick." Having admitted her, taken her history, and aspirated her abdomen, he is extra-concerned. But because she no longer needs close monitoring and is not receiving special treatment, I veto that suggestion and tell him to transfer her to the intermediate care unit, a small, three-bed facility in a neighboring ward, where extra nursing care is available. He turns to me with a stunned expression, perplexed that I could be so heartless (or stupid). His face finally relaxes when Ian Trent-Johnson pats him on the shoulder and says, "It's OK; she'll get good care there." Clearly, Ian inspires confidence among the younger residents; I am glad we agree on this one. I make a mental note to give the beginning housestaff a briefing on how the ICU should be used, only for the super-sick.

Our other new patient, Albert Monroe, is super-sick, in a dangerous state of shock because of a medical error. He is forty-seven years old and a long-term user of heroin and other intravenous drugs. He has been at SFGH on one of the medical wards for two weeks for treatment of suspected osteomyelitis—a serious infection of the bones. Three years ago, he tested positive for HIV infection, and since then he has developed AIDS with its common accompaniments: Pneumocystis carinii pneumonia, a fungus infection of his esophagus, and, most recently, a bloodstream infection with Mycobacterium avium complex, a cousin of the germ that causes tuberculosis.

Mr. Monroe was started on the usual treatment for osteomyelitis with a synthetic penicillin administered intravenously. Because he has used heroin and other intravenous drugs for decades, virtually all the accessible veins near the surface of his body are obliterated by scarring and clotting, and it was impossible to find a vein in which to give him the antibiotic. His treatment in the ward had to be interrupted until he could be taken to the operating room where surgeons implanted a catheter in one of the veins deep within his chest.

After the operation, he was started on the same intravenous penicillin derivative he had received earlier. At the end of the standard thirty-minute infusion, he complained of feeling "superwarm," and the skin all over his body turned bright crimson, an obvious allergic reaction. Luckily, he responded nicely to treatment with antihistamines. Later, though, someone gave him another injection of the same penicillinlike antibiotic! He experienced a similar reaction, but this time his blood pressure dropped and he had to be transferred to us for treatment of deep shock.

When we see him, he is less light-headed and prostrate than he was when he arrived in the ICU. He still complains that his skin is "boiling," and, to maintain satisfactory oxygenation, he must breathe air enriched with extra oxygen through a mask. Also, he continues to need a powerful muscle-constricting drug administered intravenously to increase the tone of the lax layer of smooth muscle in his arteries and restore his blood pressure to normal. Organs fail and people can die when their blood pressure is too low, so we use these constricting medications, called "pressors," in the ICU all the time. Mr. Monroe's skin looks flushed and feels hot, and abnormalities in his chest x-ray suggest that he is having a reaction in the blood vessels of his lungs entirely similar to the flushing we see in his skin. We continue his supportive care.

Allergic reactions vary greatly. The kind Albert Monroe is having, "anaphylactic shock," is undoubtedly the most dangerous and can be lethal if not properly and promptly treated. Once an allergic reaction to a medication occurs, we tell the patient and document the event in his or her medical record. In general, the culprit drug is to be forevermore avoided. Inevitably, there are exceptions to this rule, depending on the severity of the illness, the availability of alternative drugs, and the type of reaction that occurred. When an order to change a medication is written in a patient's chart, that message must be picked up by the nurse, entered into the schedule of treatments kept at the bedside, transmitted to the pharmacy, and finally implemented when the time arrives. Errors or delays can occur during any one of these steps, but we never learned exactly what happened with Mr. Monroe. Molly Wolford, our head nurse, talked to the head nurse on the ward to find out what went wrong—and to let the staff know they almost killed him.

It's time to have another talk with Truman Caughey's mother. Mr. Caughey, one of our two patients with asthma and chronic obstructive pulmonary disease, has made further progress with our efforts to liberate him from the ventilator and is getting close to being extubated. "You remember from our previous conversations, and you can see for yourself, that Truman is having a terribly rough time. That tube has been in his windpipe now for five weeks, despite all the strong medicines we have given him. This means that his lungs are severely and permanently damaged; they can't get much better. Even so, it looks as though it will be safe enough to take the tube out soon. But the tube should not be reinserted no matter what, even if his breathing failure returns, because his lung disease is not reversible. Putting the tube back will just prolong his misery. If Truman is going to die, it should happen without the added torment from the tube."

Although she and her son have not talked about heroic treatment and death, she agrees. "I guess that's what Truman would want," she says hesitantly. I breathe a sigh of relief and sympathy. I am not convinced, however, that she truly understands that his death is a real possibility, nor that this is the right way to proceed. We cannot ask Truman what he wants us to do because he has not begun to respond to questions or to simple commands even though we have lightened his sedation. I have begun to fear he has suffered brain damage from lack of oxygen during one or more of his many episodes of acute respiratory failure.

Truman Caughey demonstrates another serious pitfall in the use of heavy sedation in the ICU. Because the patient cannot talk or communicate in any fashion when drugged, there is no way to ask what is going on in his mind, and it is impossible to conduct a neurologic examination to determine if the brain is receiving and processing signals normally.

The only way to find out is to stop the medications and see what develops as they wear off. Although some patients wake up disturbingly slowly, others do not wake up at all or only partially, because undetected brain injury, usually from lack of oxygen but occasionally from a stroke, has occurred while they were in a drug-induced coma. Something of this sort seems to have befallen Mr. Caughey.

Similar issues surround Howard McVicker, the much older asthmatic with underlying lung disease, whom we extubated yesterday morning. About 6:00 in the evening, he suddenly became short of breath and started to wheeze heavily. Fortunately, he responded to additional inhaled antiasthma medications (bronchodilators). He was also gently sedated: this can be dangerous, but Ian Trent-Johnson chose to do it because he was convinced, as were we all, that anxiety was contributing to Mr. McVicker's attacks. We usually withhold sedatives during an asthma attack unless the patient is intubated. This is because asthmatics need forceful signals from their brains to sustain their labored efforts to breathe. Depressing the brain with sedatives diminishes those signals and can be fatal.

This morning Mr. McVicker looks wretched; he is disoriented, hallucinating, and expressing paranoid ideas. "They were trying to kill me; they were just here," he manages to utter in his gravelly postextubation voice. I make the diagnosis of ICU psychosis, and ask what medications he is receiving. "Lots," says the resident: three kinds of medicines to dilate constricted air passages (bronchodilators), a powerful antiinflammatory-antiasthmatic drug (methylprednisolone), four different narcotic-sedatives and an antidepressant (fentanyl, propofol, lorazepam, midazolam, and haloperidol), and an acid-suppressor to protect his stomach against the development of ulcers (cimetidine). At other times, Mr. McVicker has received a stool softener, a diuretic, and multivitamins. Of his ten regular drugs, the corticosteroid methylprednisolone, the antiulcer drug cimetidine, and the narcotic fentanyl are the most likely cause of his toxic psychosis.

Mr. McVicker's wife is with him when we make rounds. I have not met her before because she works during the day, Monday through Friday, and can come to the hospital only at night during weekdays. I am relieved that he is not alone. I review his clinical course with her, emphasizing the fact that he is gravely ill and that the new psychosis is a serious setback. She says that the nurses and other doctors have told her the same thing. She adds, "Howard has had several bad episodes before, but he's always pulled through." She seems to have a lot of faith in us. I worry that she is in for a bitter disappointment.

All drugs cause toxic side effects: there is not a single exception to this clinical maxim. There are differences among drugs only in the frequency with which they produce adverse reactions and in what the reactions are. Howard McVicker's drug-induced psychosis is particularly unwelcome because it contributes to his agitation and uncontrollable behavior, and because it means we need to stop or decrease some of his medications, which means risking the emergence of the abnormalities these medications are supposed to treat or prevent.

Several times after we made rounds yesterday morning, Constancia Noe had episodes of a dangerous racing of her heartbeat, "ventricular tachycardia," an ineffectual irregularity accompanied by a drop in blood pressure. They were finally controlled after trials of increasingly powerful medications. But even while the chaotic heart rhythm was threatening her, an offsetting miracle occurred: her respiratory status improved. So we held back the sedatives and briefly tried to see if she could breathe on her own. To our astonishment and gratification, she did well. Leaping at the opportunity, we removed the breathing tube about noon.

Amid general rejoicing at her return to consciousness, she was visited yesterday afternoon by twenty-nine members of her extended family, with whom she could communicate in a hoarse voice or by writing. Pauline Victoria did up her long black hair, and to me she looked like Violetta in the last act of La Travi-

ata, pale and beautiful. Babies were held up for her to see, and small children waved to her through the window of her room. Later that evening, after her family had left, Ian Trent-Johnson had a quiet talk with her and learned that she did not want the endotracheal tube reinserted if her breathing should worsen again, nor did she want to be resuscitated if her heart stopped beating. Ian called me at home, and I issued the order to respect her decision. During the night, she became unconscious, then deeply comatose.

She died shortly before we started ward rounds, and her grieving father and a tearful sister, who, with a pretty oval face, dark eyes, and jet-black hair, looks a lot like Mrs. Noe, are still in her room when I enter the ICU. I give them my condolences. To myself, I say, "so young, so much to live for. Another victim of drug addiction. What a waste."

I know that Constancia Noe's short life was checkered and perhaps even disreputable (people hinted that she had been a prostitute), but it meant something that she was never abandoned by her family. I have no idea what rekindled her residual life-forces and allowed her to wake up, albeit transiently, while by rights she should have continued dying. It's a motif novelists and composers love, and I have seen less striking examples a few times before—always among victims of tuberculosis. This phenomenon of a last-minute revival of energy is dramatically portrayed, historically, in the death of Charlotte Brontë's sister Anne, who, moribund from tuberculosis, rose from her deathbed, took a train to her favorite place on the seashore, where she drove a donkey cart on the sand, admired a beautiful sunset, and died in her hotel the following afternoon.[2]

Many patients in the ICU die quietly without a struggle of any sort. Sometimes, part of the tranquillity is chemically induced by morphine or other sedative drugs, but Mrs. Noe did not receive these at the end. I have seen patients who start out awake and alert, as she was Saturday evening, in whom a kind of peaceful indifference mercifully takes over, accompanied by a pervasive somnolence. At times, this state of near unresponsiveness may be provoked or amplified by a recognizable metabolic abnormality, because the kidneys, liver, or other vital organs are not functioning properly. At other times this tranquillity just seems to happen without reason. In such cases, I must admit, we rarely look for one, and are grateful when people die so peacefully.

I wish that such a peaceful death would come for our ninety-five-year-old patient, Hanako Furukawa, who remains deeply unconscious. I hope she is unaware of the endotracheal tube that remains at the behest of her children. We still lack a definite diagnosis, but the neurology consultants think she probably had a huge stroke, which fits the clinical picture better than anything else. The pneumonia we discovered yesterday is worse in both lungs. However, we have made good progress in eliminating her need for machine-assisted breathing. We now elect to take the tube out and transfer her to a regular ward. I write in my note that she should not be reintubated or brought back to the ICU.

Mrs. Furukawa left our ICU shortly after rounds as I had ordered. Later that afternoon, when she began to worsen, another discussion was held with her four children about how aggressive her care should be. By then the gravity and hopelessness of the situation had sunk in, and they agreed with our recommendations not to reintubate her for respiratory failure or to resuscitate her heart when it stopped. She remained in a deep coma and died the next day. Some deaths you'd like to have back, so life could start over again. But I don't feel that way about Mrs. Furukawa's. So far as we can tell, she has had a perfectly satisfactory ninety-five years. Now it is over, her life at its ordained end.

Hugh Martini, whom we saw for the first time yesterday with suspected pneumocystis pneumonia and AIDS, is gratifyingly stable. He is maintaining his blood oxygen in a reasonable range while breathing large quantities of added oxygen. He still gasps noticeably for breath between words as he stammers,

"I'm . . . feeling . . . better," and obviously he would rather not talk. But I judge he is holding his own: before we disturbed him, he was calmly sitting in bed reading the Sunday New York Times Book Review. *His temperature remains normal, and his chest x-ray has not worsened. There is nothing more to do except to support him vigorously until tomorrow morning, when we find out if our diagnosis is correct.*

Except when I really do not want to be disturbed, I leave the door to my office on one of the medical corridors open as an invitation to residents and students to drop in. And they do, even when I am not the attending physician of the month, to ask questions, talk about a patient, or show me an x-ray. Just after lunch, in comes Dr. Shirley Avery, one of our best first-year residents. "Can I talk to you?" she asks, sliding into a chair before I can reply. "I know you've been here a long time," she says (something I do not need to be reminded of), "so this has probably come up before." Before I can ask what, she goes on. "This is my second month at 'The General,' and almost all my patients have been losers. In the ICU alone, of my five patients, three were drunks and two were junkies. Two signed themselves out against my advice, and one has already been back to the ER twice. They're all trying to kill themselves. What's the point? Why are we doing this?"

I'm used to this question and have a prepared speech: "When you became a physician, you made a commitment to take care of people who need your help—all of them, not just those you deem worthy of your attention. You are right, San Francisco General is a very special hospital, and some of our patients make it special. I have been putting alcoholics and addicts back on the streets for nearly forty years. But what's the alternative? Are you going to not treat them and allow them to die because you disapprove of their habits? Many of these people are victims of social bad luck, not always of their own making. And as you have seen, once caught in the cycle, it's difficult to break out. These people need our help, and we must go on giving it to them. Every now and then, we have a brilliant success."

"It's a waste of time and money," Shirley contends, "my time and taxpayers' money."

That obliges me to reaffirm what I have already said: "We care for these people because we're doctors and that's our job." I add, "You are not the first person to feel this way; it's ubiquitous. But don't be judgmental. It won't help your patients, and it will drive you crazy. Concentrate on their medical problems, not their life-styles. Compassion is vital, both for your patients' medical illnesses and for their emotional reactions to them. You have to allow for ignorance, language barriers, responses you don't understand, and mistrust of physicians in general and you in particular. Feelings such as yours, dislike and disapproval, distort your thinking and affect your clinical decisions. Replace your negative thoughts with sympathy and empathy. You will be an even better doctor and your patients will benefit from it."

After Shirley sulks off, unpersuaded by these Pollyanna sentiments, I reflect on the many times I have had this conversation, in one form or another. Repetition may explain why my message now sounds more sanctimonious than originally intended, but for me it is still true. SFGH is one of a diminishing number of municipal hospitals that serve a typical inner-city population. We certainly do differ from private community hospitals: many of our ICU patients are young, desperately poor, members of racial or ethnic minorities, and suffering from one of the complications of epidemic inner-city disease—alcoholism, drug addiction, HIV infection, and mental illness. The ICUs of private hospitals, in contrast, are filled with patients who are apt to be decades older, middle-class, Caucasian, and compliant, and who are typically stricken with diseases of the elderly such as heart failure, strokes, and cancer. Making the resources of the ICU available to young victims of social deprivation holds at least the potential for a better outcome and longer future than is the case in treating older persons with an irreversible fatal disease or, at best, an intractable chronic condition. It does not always work out this way, but the possibility is always there.

When I am attending, I worry intensely and constantly about my charges, every one of them. How did Rosalie Larragasada become homeless, and where will she live when she leaves here? What are the roots of Truman Caughey's anxiety and Howard McVicker's psychosis? Will the bookish and talented Hugh Martini get at least a few more years of comfortable life? Should I have told Constancia Noe's family she had AIDS, even when it turned out they knew? My concerns, however, are focused much more on the clinical issues than on the societal handicaps that brought them on. I can help with the former but not the latter. As Shirley said as she was leaving, "It can get very frustrating." It certainly can. But that's no reason to give up; once in a while, someone's life turns around.

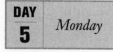

DAY 5 *Monday*

A regular part of most training programs in internal medicine is Morning Report, an enjoyable and popular teaching session. The time and format vary from one institution to another, but at SFGH two or three of the most interesting or difficult newly admitted patients are discussed by the chief of medicine, or sometimes by invited specialists, and all the residents who are free to participate. Morning Report is held every weekday morning in the chief's spartan office, where there are no chairs and only about thirty feet of couch space along three of its walls; many residents have to sit on the floor, and latecomers stand in the doorway. Plenteous coffee helps compensate for the cramped quarters. The meeting begins at 9:30 A.M., when our rounds are supposed to be over, but if the ICU is as busy as it has been since the first of the month, with a total of six or seven patients each day, our residents get tied up making rounds and cannot get to report.

Today, however, should be different. The ICU census is now down to five. Only one patient is new, and Truman Caughey, Hugh Martini, and Albert Monroe are quietly getting better; only Howard McVicker has failed to improve. We should finish early this morning, and the

48

third-year residents should get to Morning Report at last, and on time besides.

◼

Our only new patient, Edward Ramsey, is a sixty-two-year-old husky roofing contractor from Reno. After his wife's death two years ago, he has spent nearly every weekend visiting his daughter and two grandchildren in San Francisco. Yesterday, while bending over to admire the two-year-old, he abruptly began to vomit bright red blood into her crib and to experience excruciating, crushing pain, just over his heart. His son-in-law drove him to SFGH, where he told the doctors, "A load of bricks is throttling my chest." He added that for two or three days he had been passing black-looking stools, which usually means bleeding, but he drove to San Francisco Friday evening anyway. Three years ago, his private cardiologist diagnosed mild heart failure from unexplained weakening of his heart muscle, and last year he started him on an anticoagulant medication to prevent his blood from clotting.

By the time I hear about Mr. Ramsey, he has already been transfused with two units of blood. He has also received four units of fresh plasma (blood without red cells but with all the other vital ingredients) and some vitamin K, which were given to correct the drug-induced clotting abnormality. His chest pain has disappeared and his electrocardiogram, though abnormal, shows the same changes as ones in an old record faxed from Reno. Blood specimens have been collected, and we will measure the amount of a special substance, "troponin," that normally resides within heart muscle cells but that leaks into the bloodstream when the muscle is damaged. If the levels of this specific marker of heart muscle injury are elevated, they will indicate that he has bled so much he has had a heart attack.

On entering Mr. Ramsey's room, I notice that the head of his bed is elevated, which is unusual for people who have bled a lot, who generally prefer to lie flat or with their heads down to ensure that blood flows to the brain. Noticing my puzzlement, Elisabeth Viragio, his nurse, volunteers an explanation: "Edward asked me to raise his bed just after I came on duty. He said he was suffocating and had a tremendous urge to sit up." The only abnormality I find when I examine him are some crackly noises, which sound like Rice Krispies popping, in the bottom parts of both lungs each time he breathes.

Today's chest x-ray shows that his lungs are foundering in excess fluid, undoubtedly because all the blood, plasma, and other intravenous solutions he has been given are more than his weakened heart can accommodate—which explains why he wants to sit up to breathe. Regardless of what causes shortness of breath, people nearly always breathe more comfortably when sitting up than when lying down. We agree that until we know whether he has had a heart attack and can treat his pulmonary edema, we must postpone the endoscopy of his esophagus, stomach, and duodenum to seek the site of his bleeding.

There are several specific causes of the kind of progressive heart muscle attrition that Mr. Ramsey began to develop three years ago, but none was ever diagnosed. For twelve months he has been taking an anticoagulant drug to prevent blood clots from forming on the delicate membrane lining the interior of his heart cavities, a common complication of his generic type of disease. These clots pose a serious hazard because they often fragment. When they do, the broken pieces are carried by the circulating bloodstream until they finally plug blood vessels in the organ in which they have happened to land. An obstruction to blood flow anywhere in the body is dangerous because it chokes off and kills the tissues that depend on a steady supply of oxygen and nutrients for survival; in organs such as the brain, eyes, and heart, death of even a small amount of tissue can be devastating. But taking an anticoagulant means that blood will not clot when it is supposed to, which means that otherwise minor episodes of bleeding can become life-threatening.

We are concerned that Mr. Ramsey's severe hemorrhage-induced shortage of red blood cells may have led to the death of some of his already damaged heart muscle cells, which would explain his intense strangling chest pain. Although his unchanged electrocardiogram does not support this diagnosis, the final answer must await the results of the heart-muscle injury markers, due back from the laboratory this afternoon.

Today is a big one for Truman Caughey. Although his mental status has not improved, he is ready to have his breathing tube taken out after more than five weeks of dependency on a ventilator. We review yesterday's discussion with his mother and reaffirm that, in view of the severity and irreversibility of his lung disease, we are not going to put the tube back if his breathing distress returns. I explain, "Although asthma precipitated his admission to the ICU and has been troublesome, now that it is quieting down and the sedation has been almost stopped, it is apparent that at one time or another Truman's brain was damaged."

"Oh Lord, what next!" Mrs. Caughey exclaims. Then she asks, "What could happen if Truman has another bad attack and you don't put the tube thing back?"

"We'll treat him vigorously with everything we have to control the episode. If this fails, we will give him a generous amount of morphine to make sure he does not suffer in the slightest; in this way, at least he will die peacefully."

Her whole body stiffens, maybe only now grasping the possibility that he might die. Finally she relaxes and mutters, "Go ahead."

After Mrs. Caughey goes back into her son's room and we are out of earshot in the corridor, Lynn Proctor, a trim, eager medical student speaks up. I seldom learn the names of the medical students who make daily ward rounds with me because they show up and then disappear every couple of weeks; often, too, they lurk timidly in the back of the troupe, seemingly intimidated by the portentous discussions taking place. Not Lynn, though, who has already differentiated herself by asking one sensible question after another. She has more in store this morning. "You really would NOT reintubate Truman? And giving him morphine would KILL him; you said so yourself!"

Watch out, I caution myself, gaining a few seconds to think about how to explain this. Then I say, "Mr. Caughey has been in the ICU now for more than five weeks, intubated most of the time. You weren't here to notice that when he was not heavily sedated he tried to pull his endotracheal tube out and he struggled relentlessly against the ventilator, day after day. He has clearly suffered horribly. We've done all we can and have finally made sufficient progress that we can extubate him safely, and we are going to do it right now. There's no reason to wait any longer. No, we are not going to put the tube back in, and yes, if his asthma comes back and worsens despite stepped-up aerosols and steroids, we will give him morphine and allow him to die peacefully. Without the intense terror and agonizing distress of progressive asphyxia."

"Ah-hah," she replies in an I've-caught-you tone, "that sounds like a flimsy disguise for physician-assisted execution."

"Be careful with your words," I tell her, "physician-assisted suicide or euthanasia occurs when the doctor prescribes a medication or injects a lethal substance with the precise intention of causing death."

"Isn't that exactly what you said you were going to do, just a moment ago?"

"No, not at all. What I decided and what everyone seemed to agree with, including you, I thought, was that we have won this long battle at great price in view of his considerable agony and apparent loss of brain function, but we have not won the war. That has declared itself unwinnable. So if his symptoms return and do not respond to vigorous treatment, we will not let him suffer again. Morphine will see to that. The key point is that our intent is to relieve Mr. Caughey's suffering, not to cause his death, although I agree with you that morphine may quicken it."

"What's the difference?" she snaps.

This is another discussion we frequently have with students and residents. "The difference is conceptually narrow, but ethically and legally huge. Physicians are obliged to relieve pain and suffering; it's one of our oldest and greatest moral responsibilities. We are also enjoined by our own ethical standards, as well as by the prevailing laws of the land, from deliberately killing people. But given the choice between the goal of relieving the misery of dying and the recognition that the process of providing comfort might incidentally hasten an imminent death, both society and our profession are opting strongly for palliation." Lynn looks pensive but remains silent. I don't ask what she is thinking.

While we are talking outside Mr. Caughey's room, the respiratory therapist arrives and starts to unwrap the tape that holds the endotracheal tube in place. We file in and join Mrs. Caughey to watch. I glance across the bed at Lynn and see that she is wide-eyed with apprehension and has her fingers crossed. Finally, the balloon is deflated and out comes the tube. Mr. Caughey makes one feeble cough, then continues to breathe as easily as he had before. We all stand transfixed as he takes one reassuring breath after another. It is anticlimactic but a huge relief, especially for his mother, who keeps wringing her hands and saying, "Thank you, Lord, thank you." Lynn has disappeared. Now all we can do is to continue his antiasthma medications and hope these will prevent future severe attacks.

The American Thoracic Society, among other professional organizations, has sanctioned the use in these circumstances of sedatives and painkillers like morphine, the quintessential drug with the so-called "double effect," with an official statement: "It is ethically permissible to provide sufficient medication to relieve a patient's pain and suffering arising from withholding or withdrawing life-sustaining therapy, even if the patient's death may be unintentionally hastened in the process."[1] Easing death is the beneficial trade-off for possibly hastening it, given the fact that the death is inevitable and imminent. But this did not happen to Mr. Caughey. He has escaped death—so far.

In contrast to Truman Caughey, Howard McVicker has been in the ICU "only" twelve days. If we judge from his clinical condition before he was admitted, part of his respiratory failure should be reversible. Today, though, he remains delirious, and his auditory and visual furies are continuing to bedevil him. His whole body is constantly moving, tugging repeatedly on the restraints that bind his wrists and ankles, lunging against the canvas harness now fastened around his chest and strapped to the bed, and jerking his head to stare— terrified—first at one place in his room, then quickly turning to another. "They're coming, they want me, get them out of here," he moans, over and over. He needs heavy sedation, but we know that putting him to sleep will depress his breathing and that means what we want most to avoid: intubation.

Equally worrying to me is my finding that his breathing is labored and he is wheezing loudly. His chest x-ray shows subtle abnormalities, but of the same type that have come and gone on previous films. I ask Jim Shotinger, who has the duty today, to be sure to come by tonight when Mr. McVicker's wife will be visiting him. She needs to know the situation because there is a good chance we will need to intubate him again, and soon.

I am fairly confident that Howard McVicker's hallucinations and terrifying misapprehensions are caused by one of the medications he is receiving; we have already cut back on all three possible offenders. Many patients become disoriented in the ICU, though in contrast to Mr. McVicker's case, drugs are not always the chief factor. Local surroundings and the prevailing atmosphere contribute to what we call "ICU psychosis." Although not meant to resemble prison cells, our beige-colored rooms are small, thirteen by eleven feet, which does not leave much free space around the bulky bed, bedside stand, and single visitor's chair.

Claustrophobia is intensified when the bed is hemmed in by the stainless steel poles that hold plastic intravenous infusion bags but resemble prison bars, by a ventilator the size of a small refrigerator, and by an even larger dialysis machine. Confusion is further fostered by constant illumination; bright lights are on all night, making it difficult to tell one day from the next, especially while in the penumbra of sedation. To help overcome this, we have mounted a clock on the wall facing the bed, so that patients can verify the passage of time. And each room has a television set to provide another contact with the familiar world. The rooms accommodate one patient only. Even so, privacy is impossible, owing to a large window that faces the main work area with its central nurses' station. The purpose of the window is to allow the staff to observe the patient at all times, but it also permits the reverse: the patients witness the routine bustle of nurses, doctors, and visitors coming and going, not to mention the ruckus that accompanies an emergency resuscitation or new admission. This surreal atmosphere is heightened by cyclical hissing noises from ventilators and intermittent alarms that bleep, ping, and chirp in cacophanous tones. No wonder poor Mr. McVicker is raving. Perhaps the most astonishing thing about ICUs is that psychosis is not more common than it is.

Hugh Martini, the patient we treated over the weekend for suspected pneumocystis pneumonia and AIDS, has had another quiet twenty-four hours. One hour before rounds he had a sputum induction, a simple procedure in which the patient inhales a fine mist of concentrated salt solution for about five minutes. After the droplets settle in the lungs, they promote the flow of secretions and provoke coughing, which raises the material into the throat from which it can be expectorated and collected for examination. When we see him, Mr. Martini says, "I feel sensational, much better than yesterday," and his chest x-ray is definitely improved.

About the time we return to the ICU from the x-ray department, we receive a call from one of the technicians in the parasitology laboratory, who informs us that Mr. Martini's sputum is "loaded" with Pneumocystis carinii.

Among the many things that are not taught in medical school is how to break the news to someone that he or she has a fatal disease. With a person like Mr. Martini, smart and informed, I usually come right out with it. Besides, I have had a strong inkling that he knows what is going on, and we have made no secret about what we think he has and are treating him for. Accompanied by Ella, Jim, and Ian, I tell him, "They just called from the lab to say they found Pneumocystis organisms in the sample of sputum you coughed up this morning. You know this is what we thought you had and have been treating you for. So you're several days ahead in your treatment and responding well."

"This means I've got AIDS, doesn't it?" he asks.

"Yes, I'm afraid so," I reply, "but you know, it's not nearly as bad now as even a few years ago. Medications are getting better and better, and there's a new class of drugs in sight that looks fantastic."

At first he is petrified; then he breaks into an "I've-known-it-all-along" smile, though a rather bitter one. "I knew it because we all know what it means when you get the pneumonia. Several of my friends have had it. I just couldn't bear being tested. I guess I didn't want to know the truth, but now I do."

Because Mr. Martini has done well and is no longer in danger, we agree he can be transferred from the unit to SFGH's AIDS ward, where he will have access to outstanding counselors and support groups. There, too, he will be started on treatment for HIV infection, and plans will be made for outpatient follow-up.

Hugh Martini continued to improve, though slowly, and after four weeks he was finally discharged from SFGH. He still required oxygen and further treatment with another combination of antipneumocystis drugs. Six weeks after leaving the hospital and one month after stopping the antipneumocystis medications, Mr. Martini returned to the AIDS clinic on schedule. By then, he no longer needed oxygen, and he had gained back all the weight he had lost. He told his doctor he "felt great." On examination, however, a reddish purple nodule of Kaposi's sarcoma was found on the roof of his mouth.

Within a decade after the eruption of HIV-AIDS in the United States, the length of survival of afflicted patients had increased substantially, in large part because of improved treatment and prevention of its most important associated disease, *P. carinii* pneumonia. Yet better control of this complication did not stop the inexorable knockout of the immune system caused by ongoing HIV infection within the body. That greatly desired effect did not appear until the advent of multidrug therapy that included newly developed agents. Although these medications have transformed the usual course of HIV infection, they have to be taken on a rigorous schedule, there are many undesirable side effects, and there is a high frequency of virologic resistance. Before highly active antiretroviral therapy became available, the overriding question in patients who developed AIDS, if they survived whatever affliction struck first, was: What next and when? There were innumerable possibilities, all bad, and the next one for Mr. Martini was Kaposi's sarcoma, an unpleasant and recalcitrant malignancy.

Now, however, three years after highly active antiretroviral therapy became available, we still have patients admitted to our ICU with *P. carinii* pneumonia who, because they were never tested for HIV infection, failed to receive treatment that almost certainly would have prevented this life-threatening complication. The worst part is that most of these patients belong to "high risk" groups, gay men or drug abusers, and know they should be tested.

Last we visit Albert Monroe, our patient who developed anaphylactic shock after he accidentally received an intravenous dose of synthetic penicillin to which he was allergic. His fever has come down, and his oxygenation and chest x-ray are improving. There is nothing more to do now except to keep trying to whittle down the dose of the blood pressure–supporting medication that he continues to need, and then to make sure he remains stable without it.

Mr. Monroe stayed in the ICU the rest of the day while the dosage of the pressor was gradually tapered off. Later, he was transferred back to his original ward where he remained while completing treatment for his bone infection with a one month's course of substitute nonpenicillin antibiotics. Subsequently, in rapid order, he has had two admissions to SFGH for intractable diarrhea, worsening weakness, and progressive dementia; finally, debilitated and unable to care for himself, he was transferred to a hospice. No friends or relatives ever came to see him, but the caring staff at the hospice will make his death from AIDS less lonely. (As I write this, I agonize over our contribution to his slow, degrading death. There's no doubt that if I were he, I would prefer to have died from the anaphylactic shock of a few months ago.)

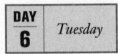

DAY 6 *Tuesday*

On Tuesdays we have Medical Grand Rounds, a formal didactic presentation of a medical topic, usually given by a member of the local faculty, but sometimes by a visiting professor from another medical school. Grand Rounds, as the name conveys, is the main event of the week in many academic institutions, where it is still conducted as in a painting by Rembrandt: all the faculty are there, sitting formally in the first few rows—although now without the dark robes and red velvet hats. Behind them are all the medical housestaff and students assigned to the medical service. The audience also includes dozens of practicing physicians from the community.

It is too bad that Grand Rounds are not such a major event at SFGH, where the sessions are held in a large, unfriendly auditorium in an adjacent building. Rain is a serious deterrent to attendance, but even on sunny days many faculty do not feel obliged to attend, and participation by the housestaff and students is desultory. I am as guilty as others of letting the old tradition slide. I rarely show up when I am attending in the ICU because I am seldom finished by 11:30 A.M., when Grand Rounds start. Today, even though we have two new exceedingly ill patients, I will interrupt my work on my notes and go because a "visiting fireman," a leading figure in the study of infectious disease, is talking about "New Antibiotics," a subject we have to keep up with.

■

I had already heard a little about today's first patient from the residents I ran into when I went into the department office to get a cup of coffee about thirty minutes before starting ward rounds. Once we convene in the ICU, I learn the whole story. Alfredo Fiorelli is a twenty-eight-year-old homeless man who has several drinks every day, and who jauntily admits that he celebrates the first day of each month (and often several days in between, it turns out), by giving himself an intravenous injection of speed. "I like to start the month on a high note," he says. "Speed," one of the popular names for methamphetamine (the other is "crank"), is a strongly addicting mental and physical stimulant. Mr. Fiorelli had greeted the beginning of the present month in his usual fashion but awakened the next day with more than his ordinary aches and pains. Subsequently, the discomfort worsened and seemed to localize in his lower back, buttocks, and rectum. Yesterday morning, when he could no longer sit down because of agonizing pain, and his legs became numb, he came to SFGH.

When an emergency department doctor first examined him, the only abnormalities he could find were fever, tenderness over his prostate gland during the rectal examination, and a high white blood cell count. A neurologist thought Mr. Fiorelli might have an abscess adjacent to his lower spinal cord, but special x-ray studies showed that the suspected region was normal. The surgeons then checked him and confirmed the presence of a tender prostate gland. They recommended a CT examination of his abdomen and pelvis, which proved informative: there are at least two large abscesses in his prostate and possible abscesses in his liver and small intestine. In addition, he has multiple abnormalities in both lungs. Worse, while he was in the x-ray department having the CT scan, his blood pressure dropped so much that by the time he was transferred to us he was in severe shock.

This morning, he requires increasing intravenous infusions of first one and then two powerful pressor drugs to support his blood pressure. Today's chest x-ray has worsened and now shows widespread marked pulmonary edema. We have him breathing as much oxygen as we can supply through a mask, just to maintain a barely satisfactory level of oxygen in his bloodstream. Two separate cultures of his blood, which were obtained only a few hours ago in the emergency department, are already growing a bacterium that appears to be a Staphylococcus. *Definitive identification will take another day.*

Our working diagnosis is circulatory collapse (shock) from widespread bloodborne staphylococcal infection, a common complication of intravenous drug abuse. We think there is a good chance that Alfredo Fiorelli also has infection of his heart valves. Even though he was started on one of the best possible antibiotics for *Staphylococcus* within minutes of his arrival in the emergency department, his shock is worsening. The urologists are concerned about the accumulated pus in his prostate gland, rightly so—but in my opinion overly so. They have scheduled him for surgery tomorrow to drain the abscesses. Because I am the attending physician, they need my permission to go ahead. Right now, I wouldn't give it; I don't believe he could survive an operation. I'll have to see how he is in the morning.

The second new patient is Richard Spencer, who came in yesterday bleeding profusely. He is a fifty-year-old chronic alcoholic who has had five previous admissions to SFGH, all for upper gastrointestinal hemorrhages. The latest of these was only four days ago, when he refused to have any diagnostic procedures and signed himself out of the hospital against the advice of his physicians. He obviously has cirrhosis of the liver, possibly due to his heavy drinking, but his blood tests reveal active hepatitis B and hepatitis C, well-known causes of cirrhosis. Even more alarming, four months ago, he had a CT study of his abdomen that led to the presumptive diagnosis of liver cancer, a common complication of cirrhosis, especially when caused by chronic hepatitis C infection.

He did agree to fiberoptic endoscopy yesterday afternoon. We found large bleeding esophageal varices, the same kind of bulging fragile veins that Mrs. Washington bled from on Day 1. Mr. Spencer's varices were injected with a congealing substance in an unsuccessful effort to sclerose the vessels and stop the hemorrhage. The problem was compounded, as is often the case in patients with severe liver disease, by failure of his blood to clot normally. The surgeons saw him last night and quite correctly said they would never take him to the operating room. "He wouldn't make it off the table."

When we examine him this morning he has already received six units of blood and three units of fresh plasma to replace the missing clotting factors. His belly is enormous, and his liver feels like a huge granite boulder. His chest x-ray shows that his lungs are flooded with pulmonary edema, undoubtedly due to all the intravenous fluids.

Richard Spencer is bleeding to death, and something needs to be done fast. One way of controlling hemorrhaging varices is to stanch them by passing a large-bore tube encircled with two big balloons down the esophagus into the stomach. First, the balloon at the tip is inflated and the tube cinched up in the stomach; then the other balloon, located in the lower esophagus, is inflated to compress the bleeding vessels. This messy procedure requires protective intubation to make sure that blood and liquids do not overflow into the windpipe and drown the patient. The presence of the two tubes, which are often left in place for several days, is odious unless the patient is deeply sedated.

Another way of possibly controlling hemorrhage from esophageal varices is to use a fluoroscope and guide a long flexible catheter through the venous system from the neck into one of the veins draining the liver. With the catheter properly positioned, an expandable plastic tube is extruded and implanted within the substance of the liver to create a "shunt," a vascular short-circuit that redirects blood through the tube instead of the varices. Using high-frequency sound waves to display his internal anatomy, we perform an ultrasonographic study to determine that Mr. Spencer is a "suitable candidate" for the short-circuiting procedure.

Accompanied by Ian Trent-Johnson, I proceed to describe the two options to Mr. Spencer, first alone and then with his son present. The son is an im-

peccably groomed and sharply dressed man about twenty-five years old. I tell Mr. Spencer in several different ways that without one of the procedures he is likely to die soon. Ian with his usual thoughtfulness adds, "Having that big tube down your gullet is pretty horrendous and it only buys time, but the approach with the catheter is easier and the benefits are long-lasting. We have had excellent results here, and so have others. I read up on it last night."

Mr. Spencer, although extremely sick, is perceptive and appears capable of making a reasoned decision. "I know what's going on," he says. "Leave me alone. I don't want anything." We go over it again, to be sure he has understood.

We turn to his son. He nods and replies, "It's Dad's choice, he knows what's best for him." He does not, at least in front of us, try to persuade his father to accept treatment.

The concept of patient autonomy, or the right to medical self-determination, is now widely accepted and generally applied in the United States. This ethical advance is bringing to a close the extended era of medical paternalism, the time when physicians such as Sir William Bradshaw in Virginia Woolf's *Mrs. Dalloway*, acting like gods, knew and did what they alone thought best for their patients. Nevertheless, implementing the concept of autonomy is sometimes made difficult because either patients or physicians do not fully understand their roles and may be unwilling or unable to accept and undertake their responsibilities.

There is no doubt about what our obligations are to Richard Spencer. He is awake and alert, knowledgeable and informed about his disease and its prognosis. If he does not want the kind of aggressive care we are prepared to offer, so be it. In many ways, his choice seems wise, because the chance of a successful long-term outcome is not good, and substantial misery is involved with either of the two procedures. Moreover, if he turns out to have liver cancer as suspected, he is absolutely doomed, because a liver transplant is out of the question.

We accept his decision without argument, also, because most of us would make exactly the same one. His son helps considerably by compassionately supporting his father's acceptance of imminent death. His son's presence eases the situation in another way. When an attending physician writes a "do not intubate or resuscitate" order (that is, an order to let the patient die), the physician is obliged to inform the family. It is much easier for them to understand the reasons for such a fateful decision when they have helped to make it.

After Mr. Spencer made his choice to let nature take its course, he received no further blood or plasma and was quickly transferred out of the ICU. He died about four hours later. His son remained with him to the end, then collapsed in a torrent of tears just after his father's death.

We received the results of the studies for heart muscle injury on Edward Ramsey yesterday afternoon. He most assuredly has had a heart attack. As soon as we learned this, we gave him more diuretics to get rid of the extra fluid he had already received and to allow us to transfuse an additional four units of blood. We wanted to increase the number of his circulating red blood cells to a higher and safer range than it had been in the morning before we knew about the test results. We certainly did not want him to have another heart attack if he bled again.

When we visit him today, he is sprightly and speaks only of "getting out of here" and going to his daughter's home "to see Leah and Stephen." Clearly, he is preoccupied with his grandchildren: he has talked to them by telephone several times. I hope his devotion does not lead him to do something rash, like sign himself out of the hospital prematurely.

He is not dissuaded when I tell him, "You've had an alarming hemorrhage plus a serious heart attack." Fortunately, all the plasma and vitamin K he has received have restored the ability of his blood to clot almost normally. Although he has had no further episodes of chest pain and has responded well to the di-

uretics, today's chest x-ray shows persistent pulmonary edema from the trans-fusions we gave him yesterday. We decide to keep him another day.

The reason Edward Ramsey had a heart attack during his brisk gastro-intestinal hemorrhage was straightforward: he had bled so much that there simply was not enough blood in his vascular system to allow his heart, which was already abnormal and striving to keep his blood pres-sure up, to maintain the circulation of life-preserving oxygen. When low blood pressure—shock—occurs, the body's protective instincts redirect what blood flow there is to preserve perfusion of the two most vital or-gans, the heart and brain, by restricting blood flow to the rest of the body. But when blood pressure falls too low, even that mechanism fails. Mr. Ramsey's severe crushing chest pain was his heart muscle shrieking for the oxygen that his circulation was unable to supply to it. This kind of heart attack, a "myocardial infarction," is common and afflicts about one and a half million Americans each year. Usually, though, these attacks occur in persons whose coronary arteries, the blood vessels that supply oxygen and nutrients to the heart, are narrowed, clogged, and hardened by arteriosclerosis. We know that Mr. Ramsey's coronary arteries ap-peared normal, at least when examined by special x-ray studies three years ago. Probably some of his diseased heart muscle, laboring as val-iantly as it could to sustain a life-preserving blood pressure, died because it required more oxygen than his beleaguered circulation could provide.

Truman Caughey, our possibly brain-damaged patient with severe asthma and chronic lung disease, whom we extubated yesterday morning with great trepi-dation, is doing amazingly well. Further good news is that his depressed brain function has improved, albeit slightly. When I ask him to squeeze my hand dur-ing my examination this morning, he does so. Later in the day, the last of the intravenous sedative drugs will be discontinued, and he will be transferred to our intermediate care unit. His mother continues to thank the Lord (and point-edly not the staff at SFGH) for what she considers a miraculous outcome. But I am not sorry for having laid it on so heavily when I told her that he could die after the tube was removed, because he very well still might. She should remain prepared for this possibility.

In contrast, our fears about Howard McVicker's worsening asthma have come true. Right after we saw him on rounds yesterday morning, his breathing became more and more labored until, finally, he was in profound respiratory distress. Ian Trent-Johnson asked me to check him again after lunch, and I agreed, reluctantly, with Ian and the respiratory therapist that he had to be reintubated.

On rounds this morning we decide to keep him sedated and mechanically ventilated another day to allow his respiratory muscles to rest up from their strenuous workout yesterday. Tomorrow, we will lighten the sedation and try again to extubate him. I will set up a meeting with his wife to explain that the likelihood of helping him is diminishing with each failure to breathe on his own. It had at first seemed that Howard McVicker would improve, but his lungs are resisting our best efforts. His chronic obstructive pulmonary disease is unquestionably severe, and, so far at least, his "asthma"—the reactive shutdown of his air passages—has proved irreversible.

Medical Grand Rounds is a big disappointment. The lecturer, the worst kind of arrogant academic, talks mainly about the potential of antibiotics that are in the commercial "pipeline" of the future, each one illustrated by detailed drawings of its three-dimensional chemical structure, which only a few of the biochemically oriented infectious disease experts understand. It is like a technical ad for the pharmaceutical industry, something all doctors get too much of as it is. I begin to suspect he is on the payroll of one of the drug companies. We clinicians are all baffled. He hardly speaks at all about what most of us have come to hear: how should we best use the antibiotics that we already have, including new ones that we are not very familiar with.

I tell one of my faculty colleagues as we are leaving that from now on I'm not sitting in the second row as I always try to do. That talk was terrible, and I have my notes to write. I desperately wanted to leave, I confide, but it was too embarrassing to walk out.

My friend says, "I'm just not going to come anymore."

One of the most popular, and certainly the best-attended, of the regular organized teaching sessions, the Morbidity and Mortality Conference, more simply "M & M," is held every Wednesday at noon. The purpose of M & M is to sharpen diagnostic acumen and improve clinical proficiency by reviewing confusing or complex cases, analyzing causes of complications, usually those that might have been prevented, and examining how and why patients died, especially if death was unexpected. For young doctors it's a good opportunity to sort out the problems and anxieties that accompany unforeseen disasters and to emphasize the importance of one of the fundamental truths of medicine: *first, do no harm.* An attractive feature of the meeting is the serving of pizza and soft drinks. The housestaff get free meals in the hospital cafeteria anyway, but this lunch is especially convivial, albeit an odd occasion for conviviality.

Usually two patients are discussed in some detail in a kind of game-show format. The responsible second-year resident summarizes the patient's complaints and findings and gives the results of the initial round of laboratory tests; any early x-rays are shown by a member of the radiology faculty. Next, the chief of medicine asks one of the other residents, who does not know the solution, to formulate a differential diagnosis and to suggest a strategy to sort out the true answer from among the possibilities. Subsequent clinical events and test results are described, and the inquisition goes on. Representatives of various specialty divisions and surgical or other services are there to comment. There is nearly always an answer to a diagnostic dilemma—a positive bacteriological study, a critical x-ray finding, or a definitive laboratory test result. When pathologists are in the audience there is an anatomic denouement too: either colorful microscopic sections of a biopsy projected on the screen or, better yet, all or parts of organs from an autopsy, fresh or pickled, that reveal the give-away abnormalities. I have noticed that not even a pus-filled gall bladder or hemorrhagic brain seems to disturb the consumption of pizza.

The ICU is always a rich source of material for M & M. Two days ago, the chief resident, who organizes the sessions, asked me whether Albert Monroe and his anaphylactic shock would be suitable. I readily agreed, but it won't happen. That presentation has been preempted by a new case of "meningitis," an often deadly infection of the delicate membranes surrounding the brain, which the chief of medicine thinks transcends all others in importance, and which has been the subject of a lot of his research.

The first of our four new patients proves to be an old friend to me and many on the unit. She was recently hospitalized here for nearly four months and left SFGH only twelve days ago, just a week before our present rotation began. Moreover, I was the attending physician in the ICU during the first three weeks of her long stay here. Claudia Jonson is a seventy-two-year-old transvestite who is known for her mane of bright yellow hair and her extravagantly colored flowing dresses. Although wheelchair-bound, she picks up extra money and enjoys playing the barrel organ near one of the local tourist hangouts. About four months ago, for reasons we never fully understood, she fell over backward and struck her head on the sidewalk. The barrel organ toppled over on her chest, fracturing several ribs and the collar bone on the left. In the emergency department, a tube had to be inserted into her chest to drain blood that had accumulated in her left chest cavity.

This part went smoothly, but thereafter she had one complication after another. The first was the development of kidney failure—uremia—from an enlarged prostate and a huge stone that nearly filled her bladder. Her kidney function worsened to the extent that she needed dialysis.

As if this weren't enough, the second complication was respiratory failure, precipitated by the injury to her chest but superimposed, as in so many of our patients, on underlying chronic obstructive pulmonary disease, emphysema, and bronchitis. Her breathing became so impaired she required intubation and a ventilator.

And there was a third complication: recurrent episodes of irregular heartbeat, during which her heart rate would speed up and her blood pressure would drop. This problem was easier to solve than the others; it was finally corrected by surgical implantation of an artificial pacemaker, a device that triggers a regular heartbeat when the heart's natural rhythm becomes chaotic.

We suspected a fourth complication—impaired brain function resulting from the head injury—but this was impossible to assess accurately because of her need for pain-relieving medications and sedatives. When it became clear she would need prolonged breathing assistance, we had the surgeons perform a "tracheotomy," an operation in which a hole is made into her windpipe and a tube inserted to connect her to a ventilator. This procedure allowed us to take out the endotracheal tube, which damages the vocal cords when left in place longer than a few weeks.

In addition to Ms. Jonson's complicated medical problems, there was a feeling problem: we had all grown fond of her. At first, everyone caring for her— housestaff, nurses, and myself included—had to learn to call her "her" rather than "him." On rounds at the beginning of her long hospitalization, "Mr. Jonson" was sometimes used, and references to "him/his/he" prevailed. But it soon became clear that she wanted to be called Claudia or Ms. Jonson, and so she was, first by the nurses, then by the housestaff, and last by me. What slowed me down was the fact that I examined her every day. Once you looked under the covers, there was no doubt that, anatomically, she was a man.

After almost four months of innumerable complications, she was transferred to a private facility in the Bay Area for chronic care and weaning from the breathing machine. Soon after her arrival there, however, she had to be started on an antibiotic for yet another urinary tract infection; but the medication proved toxic to her kidneys and exacerbated her preexisting kidney failure. So, five days later, here she was, transferred back to us for resumption of dialysis.

When we see Ms. Jonson today, I cannot tell if she knows where she is or recognizes us, her old medical friends. She is almost unresponsive even to painful stimuli, her breathing is performed entirely by a ventilator through the tracheotomy, and her chest x-ray shows pulmonary edema. She needs to be seen right away by the kidney specialists about dialysis. We will also have to check with the urologists to see if anything can be done to relieve the mechanical obstructions causing her uremia.

There are a lot of repeaters in the ICU business, so déjà vu occurs over and over. But I never expected to see Claudia Jonson again. Despite her having several diseases that did not seem to bother her much (certainly not enough to have them treated), she had lived a joyful life until the accident. Then, everything started to fall apart at the same time. I remember telling the medical housestaff accompanying me on rounds shortly after her first admission the story of the "The Wonderful One-Hoss Shay," the fabulous buggy that "ran a hundred years to a day" in absolutely perfect condition and then "went to pieces all at once." But this metaphor for what Ms. Jonson's body was doing fell flat because the residents had never heard of Oliver Wendell Holmes, Senior, much less read the poem.

The fears I was trying to express in quoting Holmes were well founded, sad to say, and I have often seen them materialize. Some people grow old quietly and gradually, seemingly without being smitten along the way by any of the perils of aging. But what appears in them to be vigorous health is a sham. Aging takes its inexorable toll by the narrowing and hardening of arteries, insidious attrition of muscle bulk and strength (including the heart muscle), deterioration of protective immunologic responses, and loss of vital functions of every organ. It should not be surprising that, when a minor insult strikes such a resourceless worn-out body, like the "One-Hoss Shay" it simply falls apart. I thought this might happen to Ms. Jonson during her first hospitalization, and it very nearly did. Now she is back, once again trying to die.

A side note for those who have begun to wonder about the economics of such care: I later learned that Claudia Jonson's first three and one-half months of hospitalization at SFGH had cost $580,000. This figure does not include physicians' fees, which are not paid to the doctors but are billed to insurance, Medicare, or Medicaid, and used by the departments involved in her care: medicine, urology, surgery, ear-nose-throat, and anesthesiology. The total charges so far must be close to three-quarters of a million dollars.

Our second new patient, Bi-Ya Ng, is a seventy-two-year-old housewife who went to a private hospital yesterday evening complaining of vomiting blood and dizziness. The doctors there aspirated bright red blood from her stomach. Her hematocrit, which indicates how many red blood cells are circulating in the bloodstream, was half the normal value. She was transferred to SFGH for "further treatment" of her gastrointestinal bleeding. In hospital code, this means she does not have medical insurance or sufficient funds to pay for private care; otherwise they surely would have kept her.

We have already given her three units of blood, and she has stabilized nicely. I find myself looking closely at her. Originally a small woman, she is now even smaller because of severe osteoporosis, or bone wasting, which has collapsed several vertebras and bowed her spine forward. The deformity is so marked I wonder if she is in pain. Like Mrs. Hong last week, Mrs. Ng speaks no English, but we have no trouble communicating with her through her granddaughter, a bright university student; other grandchildren will follow her, taking shifts at the bedside. "No, Pawpaw has no pain," her granddaughter tells me. "Thank you for asking."

While we are in the x-ray department, a fiberoptic endoscopy shows two half-inch ulcers in Mrs. Ng's duodenum but no signs of bleeding. Biopsies are taken from the healthy lining of her stomach, not from the ulcerated tissue. I expect her course to be smooth enough for her to leave the ICU tonight.

Bi-Ya Ng left the unit as planned and the hospital the next day. Microscopic examination of the biopsies revealed *Helicobacter pylori*, a bacterium that infects the lining of the stomach. Only recently has this long-known microorganism been definitely linked to peptic ulcers; now ninety-five percent of duodenal ulcers and sixty-five percent of gastric (stomach) ulcers are attributable to *H. pylori* infection. Given these high percentages, it is no longer cost-effective to obtain biopsies in all patients, especially those with duodenal ulcers—they are assumed to have *H. pylori*. Since we have learned that eradicating the germ drastically reduces the rate of recurrence of peptic ulcers, the effect on patient management has been amazing. The recommended treatment of *H. pylori*-related ulcers is a two-week course of multiple antibiotics, usually with conventional antiacid therapy for four weeks. Complete and long-lasting healing occurs in nearly all cases, a superb accomplishment in treating a previously recurrent and refractory disease. Now we can actually cure most peptic ulcers.

The third new patient is a thirty-seven-year-old unemployed man, Ralph Rennes, who visits the emergency department regularly and who has had innumerable admissions to SFGH for alcoholism, including convulsions, delirium tremens, and complications of alcoholic cirrhosis of the liver. Last night, he was brought to the hospital by ambulance after being found in one of the city parks in a stupor. Laboratory studies showed his blood alcohol was 450 mg/dl (milligrams per deciliter, a standard way of reporting the concentration of many

substances in circulating blood), high enough to kill an intolerant (alcohol na-
ïve) person, but not someone as accustomed to it as he is. (The legal definition of
a drunk driver in California is the presence of a blood-alcohol level above
80 mg/dl.) Not unexpectedly, his liver was functioning poorly.

Disheveled and red-faced with the whisky redolent in his breath, he un-
leashes a fast and ugly temper and complains of a severe headache. Because he
resists my examination, I have to enlist the help of residents on each side of the
bed to hoist his upper body so that I can check his lungs in the back. While I am
trying to listen to his heart and lungs, he keeps talking and occasionally belches.
He has a greatly enlarged liver and spleen, and his trunk and arms are speck-
led with skin abnormalities characteristic of cirrhosis, called "spider angiomata"
because their long, slender vascular branches resemble daddy longlegs. But I
conclude that Mr. Rennes does not need further care in the ICU and order his
residents to transfer him to the ward.

Ralph Rennes, who is known to the SFGH medical and nursing staff
as one of our "Frequent Flyers," does not believe in clean living. Nor do
many of the other patients we have seen during the last week, who uni-
formly resist all efforts at reform and rehabilitation. Their views are reflected in the old story, which one of my gurus told me decades ago
when I was a resident in medicine, about the man who went to see his
physician because he was coughing, had no pep, and was concerned
about his increasing weight. The doctor, knowing his patient was a chain
smoker, heavy drinker, and insatiable glutton, advised him to quit smoking, stop drinking, and go on a strict diet. The worried patient thought
for a moment, and then asked, "If I manage these feats, will I live a lot
longer?"

To which the doctor instantly replied, "No, but it will seem a lot
longer!"

Today, the answer would be different. Stopping smoking, curtailing
drinking, and losing excess weight are undeniably beneficial. Purify
your life and you're likely to live longer. I told this story to Ella, Ian, and
Jim this morning while we were waiting in the x-ray department for the

radiologist to show up. Clean-living Jim volunteered that he was concerned about living too long because he dreaded the idea of being disabled from heart failure or cancer. Ian's fears turned out to be Alzheimer's disease and strokes. "Something bad will happen, you can count on that," Ella added cheerfully, "but at least you'll feel better until it does. Relax and enjoy it." As usual, she was absolutely correct. But at her age, I doubt if she is much troubled by intimations of mortality.

Our fourth new patient is Francis Zohman, a sixty-two-year-old former barber, who was transferred back to us last night from one of the medical wards. For seven years, he has suffered from refractory asthma and needs large daily doses of prednisone, a potent cortisone drug. The nurses and respiratory therapists know him because he was hospitalized a month ago for asthma that required intubation for a few days. Shortly afterward, he underwent emergency surgery for a burst colon. He had to be reintubated for the operation, and only after several stormy days was he extubated and able to leave the ICU.

He came back early this morning, sobbing and groaning with pain from another episode of colonic distention. To decrease the risk of repeat rupture, we have treated him with enemas and have inserted a long fiberoptic flexible tube through his rectum into the enlarged colon to suck out the gas. His asthma has waxed and waned throughout this admission. He had a bronchoscopy (similar to an endoscopic examination of the gastrointestinal tract, but of the lungs) two days ago in an effort to clear his bronchial tubes of thick mucus plugging his air passages and causing parts of his lungs to collapse.

The clinical situation has quieted now. When we go into his room to see Mr. Zohman, it is obvious that he has been taking large doses of prednisone for a long time. His head and neck are puffy and red, suppurating acne covers his face, a characteristic "buffalo hump" protrudes from his back, and his belly is obese with prominent bluish stretch marks marring the skin. Despite all the prednisone, I can hear faint wheezes over both of his lungs. When I listen to his abdomen for the sounds of gas moving within the intestines, medically called by the onomatopoetic term "peristalsis," the gurgles are sluggish. This morning's x-ray of his abdomen reveals less distention of the colon. "Sorry you had to come back to us," I tell him with avuncular jocularity, "but we're off to a good start." What I don't say, because it won't do him much good, is that we have a lot to worry about.

The characteristic features of severe, life-threatening asthma, as opposed to the mild, wheezing kind most people can live with fairly easily, are now well documented: frequent attacks that require emergency treatment or hospitalizations, need for large doses of cortisone-type drugs by mouth to prevent exacerbations, and previous admissions to an ICU, especially those requiring intubation. Francis Zohman has had them all. In addition, he has been in the hospital for more than a month. This alone indicates that he has not responded well to vigorous therapy, administered on schedule and under supervision, which in turn means that we have no further improved treatment program to offer. To make matters even worse, he is back in the ICU with another difficult complication, which is probably related to the medications he is receiving and, like his asthma, will probably recur. We must prepare ourselves for a long and difficult course, punctuated, as Mr. Zohman has already displayed, by frequent setbacks.

Our SFGH guest from Reno, the burly roofer Edward Ramsey, has spent a quiet twenty-four hours, and his chest x-ray is much improved. He has shaved and is spruced up in a natty bathrobe, reliable signs of well-being and high morale. All good reasons to transfer him to one of the medical wards for a brief stay before it is safe for him to return to his grandchildren.

Edward Ramsey, who was prescribed an anticoagulant for heart disease by his cardiologist, almost bled to death and suffered a heart attack as a consequence. He and Howard McVicker, who is in the throes of a drug-induced psychosis, remind us once more that even when given for precisely the right reasons, and even when taken in exactly the right amounts, medications—all of them—can be dangerous. Albert Monroe, too, nearly died from an injection of a common antibiotic, but one he should not have received after his first allergic reaction.

Alfredo Fiorelli, our patient with widespread infection who went into shock in the x-ray department thirty-six hours ago, is still in shock when we see him this morning, and is no better than when he arrived. The bacteria circulating in his bloodstream have been identified as Staphylococcus aureus, *a hostile and venomous germ; the only good news is that they do not appear to have infected his heart valves.*

Because Mr. Fiorelli remains violently ill, I decide to cancel the planned surgical drainage of the abscesses in his prostate, over the strenuous objections of the chief resident in urology, who has come to the ICU to take Mr. Fiorelli to the operating room himself. "But he's already on the schedule," the urology resident protests.

I try to explain. "You're right that those abscesses need to be evacuated as soon as possible; there's no doubt about that. But he's too sick. Trust me. His ability to tolerate an anesthetic will improve soon. It has to." I add, "We also know the prostate is only one of several sites where he has staph, and you can't drain or excise them all; the antibiotics will have to do the job for now."

"But he's already on the schedule!" is his rejoinder and only response, except a long awkward silence that I choose not to break. I lurk around protectively until the urologist leaves.

Howard McVicker, still one of two patients in the ICU with asthma and chronic lung disease (Truman Caughey was transferred out of the unit, but Francis Zohman was transferred back in), remains terribly sick. He has returned to the clinical state he was in for more than a week before our aborted effort at extubation. He continues to have intermittent episodes of agitation and restlessness accompanied by wheezing. It is impossible to tell what else is going on because he is so heavily sedated. Nothing has changed, so we keep on as we are, still hopeful but increasingly concerned.

During the afternoon, the chief resident in medicine comes to my office to tell me that she wants to discuss Alfredo Fiorelli at next week's M & M. "What did you say to Bart Reston [the urology resident I had confronted]? He went ballistic, so furious that both ears were smoking."

"All I did was to cancel the operation he wanted to carry out this morning," I replied. "Sure, let's talk about it. It'll be interesting."

Then I go to the office of the chief of urology, whom I know well and have great respect for, to get his views. He is caught between wanting to support his resident ("We really should get that pus out of there") and appreciating my understanding of Mr. Fiorelli's medical plight ("It certainly would be safer when he's not in shock"). We agree that they will put him back on tomorrow's surgical schedule and that we will all meet in the ICU at 7:30 A.M. to judge together if it is safe to go ahead with the operation.

As they say around here, Ella Andrews, our high-spirited ICU resident, "got bombed" yesterday: seven new ICU admissions, including the transfer back of a patient we had cared for briefly a few days ago. To complicate matters further, our eleven patients are spread out among three different units, which adds to the logistical difficulties. As planned, I show up at 7:30, a half hour early, to meet with the head of urology and his chief resident to decide if it is safe for Alfredo Fiorelli to have his operation. Bart Reston looks sullen, says nothing, and sticks close to his boss's side.

Apparently unaffected by her frantic twenty-four hours on call, indefatigable Ella tells the three of us that Mr. Fiorelli's high fever has been unremitting the last twenty-four hours, indicating (to no one's real surprise) that his widespread staphylococcal infection is rampant. More important from a clinical standpoint and with respect to his operability is the fact that the pressor medications have been stopped. He is no longer in shock. We all agree that now is the time to take Alfredo Fiorelli to the operating room for drainage of his prostatic abscesses. Bart Reston, now positively grinning in anticipation, tells us what's in store for

Mr. Fiorelli, who listens anxiously. "I'll insert a scope through his penis to the level of the prostate gland, locate the abscesses with a small ultrasonic probe, and incise the overlying tissue so that the pockets can empty directly into the urethra [the tube that carries urine as it flows from the bladder to outside the body]."

"Up my dick?" says Mr. Fiorelli, writhing. "You're going to shove what up my dick?"

"Only a tiny instrument, slimmer than a pencil," interjects Ella. "The one I told you about last night. To get rid of the pus."

"Oh that," says Mr. Fiorelli as he scribbles his name on the consent form with a wobbly hand. I sign the bottom of the page as a witness.

We start regular rounds in the surgical unit on the fourth floor where we see our first new patient, Joseph Schwartz, a fifty-two-year-old alcoholic, who was brought to SFGH last night by ambulance workers who had spotted him sitting in the middle of a street in the Tenderloin district. He was confused, smelled strongly of liquor, and was shivering. Apparently no one had called for help— Mr. Schwartz was simply found by a pair of paramedics from one of the city's ambulance squads, who know where to look for business, and who are often successful in finding people who might otherwise lie undiscovered for hours. In the emergency department, Mr. Schwartz's temperature was only 93.2° F. and decreased even lower, to 88.2° F., well below the normal value of 98.6° F—serious chilling of the body, known as "hypothermia." The emergency room doctors began warming him with heated intravenous fluids and several extra blankets, and sent him up to us. Ella Andrews decided to start him on three different antibiotics because there was a good chance that he had an infection and that it was disguised by the hypothermia.

Mr. Schwartz did not just warm to normal; his body temperature kept climbing. This morning, he has a high fever, 104.5° F., and pneumonia has blossomed in both lungs. Still, his treatment from now on is straightforward, and he no longer needs to be in an ICU; so we make plans to transfer

him to a medical ward later in the afternoon, where they can deal with the
pneumonia.

Joseph Schwartz started out as a typical case of dangerously low body temperature. Hypothermia, a common condition, is nearly always caused by exposure to cold weather, but it is more likely to occur when a person is wet, for damp clothes increase the rate of heat loss from the body. Hypothermia is also more likely when a person has been drinking alcohol or using drugs that impair the body's protective heat-conserving defenses. Given the types of patients we care for, we see a lot of hypothermia at SFGH. From a study carried out here several years ago, we learned that about half of our patients with the condition also had an underlying serious infection that was often undetectable at the time of admission.[1] This is why Ella Andrews started the antibiotics, and it was a smart thing for her to have done.

Mr. Schwartz warmed up nicely with simple measures, but it was only after the hypothermia had been corrected that his severe pneumonia became apparent. Moreover, his blood cultures grew *Staphylococcus aureus*, the same tough microbe that nearly killed Alfredo Fiorelli. Despite his having received optimum antibiotic treatment, Mr. Schwartz continued to have a high fever every day, and his condition failed to improve. An abdominal CT scan and other special studies to look for hidden sites of infection were recommended, but he refused further evaluation. Despite pleading and warning of death by all his doctors, he insisted on leaving the hospital, probably to resume drinking. He was supposed to receive further antibiotics from visiting nurses, but our hospital records do not show whether he did, and he has not been seen again. This is a tragedy. The man had his life to live, and his disease was probably curable.

We move around the corner from Mr. Schwartz's room to hear about Gertrude
Davies, another fifty-two-year-old alcoholic who has already been in the ICU

*for five days as a patient of the surgeons. Important parts of her story are sup-
plied by Clare Brownstein, a social worker who has been helping to care for
Mrs. Davies for many years and knows her well. She tells us that Mrs. Davies
and her husband had once owned and run a successful dry-cleaning business.
Eight years ago, after their only son had been killed in a drive-by shooting, she
started drinking and never stopped, despite several attempts at rehabilitation.*

*On the evening of her admission, she staggered into the emergency depart-
ment, obviously drunk. Dark blood blackened her sweater near the right shoulder, where a spike of her newly fractured upper arm bone (humerus) was pok-
ing through the overlying muscle, skin, and clothing. Apparently she had fallen,
an all-too-common hazard when people are drunk. Because it was suspected she
might also have injured one of her abdominal organs, she was taken to the operating room, where the surgeons made a small incision through the wall of her
abdomen so that they could check inside for blood and other signs of trauma;
nothing abnormal was found. After the abdominal exploration, while she was
still intubated and anesthetized, the bone and joint experts, the "orthopedists,"
washed the fragment of bone that stuck out of her shoulder and manipulated the
pieces to align the fracture. Then her arm was immobilized in a sling.*

*This was not the end of it. After the operation, she developed pneumonia
with respiratory failure and had to be reintubated. The incision in her abdominal wall and the hole in the skin of her right shoulder became ugly, gaping wounds. To compound the problem, laboratory tests showed worsening anemia. Because of these medical problems, responsibility for her care had been
officially transferred from surgery to medicine last night, and I see her this
morning. Her lungs now sound unpleasantly juicy and wheezy, both wounds
are wide open, and her ankles are swollen with fluid. Her chest x-rays, as we
had been warned, show patchy areas of pneumonia, her hematocrit is low and
dropping, and the concentration of albumin in her blood, an essential protein, is
decreased.*

There is no doubt about what is wrong with Gertrude Davies, but it is
problematic whether we can fix it. Because of her alcohol-induced malnutrition, she is so enfeebled that she cannot breathe by herself, and nei-

ther her fracture nor her wounds can heal. The surgeons have made a good start by giving her supplementary feedings through a tube they passed through her nose and stomach into her duodenum, and she is tolerating this nourishment well. We decide to increase the number of calories she is receiving and to increase her hematocrit by giving her two units of blood. Our plan is to fatten and strengthen her, while treating her pneumonia and wheezing to liberate her from the ventilator.

Next, we go back to the fifth floor to visit Irwin Babcock, a thirty-six-year-old man who is resolutely hooked on methamphetamine. Last week, he went on a four-day speed binge, injecting amphetamines intravenously several times a day. Last night, he again injected himself, this time using a newly purchased street mixture called "dirty crank." One hour later, he developed chills, headache, breathlessness, and dizziness. When he could no longer stand up, he called the ambulance that brought him to SFGH. In the emergency department, the physicians discovered that his blood pressure was barely detectable and started intravenous fluids. Pressor medications were added to produce a semblance of blood pressure, and he was hastily sent to the ICU.

We learn that four months ago Mr. Babcock was found, like so many injection-drug users, to have a positive blood test for HIV infection, and his CD4+ T-lymphocyte count at the time was 400 cells/μl. This meant that although he had moderate immunological devastation produced by the virus, which seeks out CD4+ T lymphocytes and selectively destroys them, he did not have AIDS, the last of the progressive stages of evolving HIV infection. AIDS occurs when the count falls below 200 cells/μl or when certain diseases are diagnosed (like Pneumocystis carinii *pneumonia, tuberculosis, or Kaposi's sarcoma). He was referred to SFGH's AIDS clinic for comprehensive treatment, but he never showed up.*

When we see Mr. Babcock, he is still in shock and now has ICU-induced pulmonary edema from excessive intravenous fluids. We add another antibiotic to enlarge the spectrum of infections covered by our treatment, because he might be infected with an unusual germ. We have no clues as to what is trying to kill him.

"Speed kills," both on the highways and when injected into the bloodstream. The collapse of Irwin Babcock's circulation suggests to us that the "dirty crank" he used was contaminated with some sort of poison. But we cannot ignore the possibility that his plummeting blood pressure and desperate condition are caused by "septic shock" from toxins released by bacteria. Septic shock or severe blood poisoning is a recurring problem in the ICU, especially in patients with HIV infection. Thus, we have no choice but to use the shotgun antibiotic approach and to hope that our scatter is broad enough to dispatch whatever microbes are pillaging his body. In these circumstances, cultures of blood usually reveal the offenders, but we will have to wait to find out.

Our next new patient, Jaime Aguinaldo, is a forty-six-year-old auto mechanic who has been in outstanding health all his life. Yesterday afternoon he suddenly vomited a large quantity of bloody material and became so dizzy he had to lie down. After he arrived in the ICU last evening, the gastroenterologists performed an emergency endoscopy in hopes of locating the source of his bleeding. What they found instead was a hugely dilated esophagus that was nearly filled with clotted blood; it was impossible for them to see anything but blood, and they were unable to locate the opening into his stomach.

He was then taken to the x-ray department, where he swallowed liquid barium sulfate, a metallic compound that shows up vividly on x-rays; the films revealed that the barium had pooled within his enormously distended esophagus and had not entered the stomach at all. His esophagus, we could see, was enlarged the length of his chest, but narrowed at its junction with the stomach in the upper abdomen.

This morning Mr. Aguinaldo has stabilized well and cannot understand what all the fuss is about. "Hey, I feel fine now," he says. "Time to go home."

He denies any problems swallowing but does admit to having to drink a little water while eating to encourage the passage of food into his stomach.

After reviewing Jaime Aguinaldo's x-rays, we know that he has an obstruction where his esophagus joins the stomach, but we do not know where all the blood came from or the exact nature of the blockage. After considerable deliberation, with opinions from surgeons and gastroenterologists, we decide to ask our anesthesiologists to intubate him in order to protect his windpipe from the entrance of liquid and to allow him to be anesthetized. When people are comatose or anesthetized, for whatever reason, we often intubate them to assist their breathing and to guard against fluid overflowing into their windpipes and lungs. Mr. Aguinaldo is at enormous risk of aspirating or, even worse, drowning, because he has accumulated so much fluid in his esophagus.

Next, the gastroenterologists will insert a small hose into his esophagus to wash out the clots and barium that fill it. When it is finally emptied, they will reendoscope him. This scheme should enable us to find out what is going on in that strangely commodious organ.

Next we go to visit forty-nine-year-old Danny Edwards, yet another heavy alcoholic and regular heroin user, who came to SFGH yesterday because of fever, cough, shortness of breath, and sharp pain in the right side of his chest. He said he had lost twenty-five pounds during the last two to three weeks. A chest x-ray showed a large amount of fluid in the right side of his chest; so after he arrived in the ICU, the admitting resident stuck a needle between his ribs and sucked back thick greenish fluid that resembled split-pea soup. Examination under a microscope showed innumerable pairs of slightly pointed bacteria interspersed among a multitude of multilobed white blood (pus) cells. Because Mr. Edwards had a serious chest infection called an "empyema," Ella Andrews started him on antibiotics and asked our surgeons to insert a chest tube to drain the quart or more of pus that remained in the right pleural cavity.

During our examination, I take time to point out and marvel with those present at Mr. Edward's extraordinary clubbing of the fingers, a classical medical finding that is seldom encountered nowadays. Clubbing, an abnormality that causes the fingertips to enlarge and look like knobby drumsticks, was first described about 400 B.C. by Hippocrates in patients, like Mr. Edwards, with purulent chronic lung disease, although there are many other causes. His morning's chest x-ray, after much of the pus was drained through the tube, shows a large region of pneumonia in the lung next to where the fluid had been.

Drug addicts and alcoholics—and Danny Edwards was both—are much more likely than otherwise healthy persons to develop bacterial pneumonia. We have learned that when abusers of any kind of substance get sick, they often take refuge in their apartments or hotel rooms, to drink or shoot up, hoping to feel better. By the time they finally arrive at the hospital, their disease is usually far advanced. Empyema, a late complication of pneumonia, is a good example.

Rosalie Larragasada, the woman with severe alcoholic cirrhosis and multiple infections, had to be transferred back yesterday evening because of brisk gastrointestinal hemorrhage. Like Jaime Aguinaldo, she had undergone emergency fiberoptic endoscopy, which revealed severe erosions of her esophagus and a deep ulcer crater in her stomach in which an artery was spurting blood. As we have already seen in patients with advanced liver disease who start to bleed, the hemorrhage persisted because her blood failed to clot normally.

Now she is receiving her eighth unit of red blood cells and her fourth unit of fresh plasma. She barely moves her arms and legs when I pinch her skin, not even when I press hard on the ridge of bone above her eye; her brain is deeply depressed. Compared with my findings just four days earlier, her skin and eyes are now bright yellow, indicating her jaundice has worsened, and her abdomen and legs have become hugely swollen with fluid.

We consult surgeons about the possibility of an operation to control the bleed-

ing. "No way," says the chief resident. "That would be physician-assisted eu-
thanasia." We also consult radiologists to see if they can thread a catheter into
the artery supplying the ulcer and then inject a gluey substance to stop her bleed-
ing. "Absolutely not," we hear, "technically impossible."

After taking in these negative replies, I assemble her team to discuss how
we should proceed. As usual, I start at the bottom and work up the ladder of
their experience. "OK, what do we do now?" I ask the first-year resident car-
ing for her.

New to these crises, he wants to continue our full-bore attack. "Let's talk to
the surgeons again," he pleads, "and keep giving her blood." I point out that she
has already received eight units of blood and four of plasma, and that our blood
bank's supply is finite. "We should intubate her and keep going," he insists.
"We've got to; otherwise she'll die."

Next I ask the second-year resident, "Do you agree? Perhaps you should start
by telling us what is wrong with her." She gets the point, and replies shrewdly,
"She has terminal liver failure." The three third-year residents nod their heads
in agreement: in reality, there is nothing more to do.

Rosalie Larragasada was bleeding to death, and there was no possibility
of stopping it. We could not talk to her because she was comatose, and
there was no family to consult about how she would want us to proceed.
I discussed the problem with the attending physician who had cared for
her the last four days on the medical service and who knew her better
than I did. We agreed that the situation was hopeless. I wrote a "do not
resuscitate" order and transferred her out of the ICU that evening. Her
coma deepened and she died early the next day.

According to legal experts and philosophers, there is no difference
between *withholding* life support from a dying patient, as we decided was
best for Rosalie Larragasada, and *withdrawing* it after it has already been
started, as I ordered done to Patrick Guzman. They are indubitably correct that the outcome is the same in both instances: death. But, like the
majority of ICU physicians, I find it much less emotionally wrenching
not to start aggressive life support than to have to call it quits after set-

ting it in motion. Though the underlying disease is the agent of death in both instances, when I give the order to stop, I assume some of the blame for that result. The difference between withholding (passive) and withdrawing (active) is not trivial to those of us who have to intervene with fate. I have often wondered—with a certain asperity—if the same legal experts and philosophers who pronounce on these issues so confidently would throw the switch to turn off the breathing machine keeping a patient alive and extinguish the minuscule, persistent remnant of that life.

The last of our new patients, Alexandra Papandreo, was intubated and transferred to the unit last night for severe respiratory failure. She is a sixty-five-year-old, newly retired, red-haired seamstress with several medical problems, including high blood pressure, chronic unexplained anemia, and old quiescent tuberculosis. She has smoked one to two packs of cigarettes daily for over fifty years. A few months before this hospitalization, she was diagnosed as having asthma; at the time, her shortness of breath and chest tightness responded well to the usual treatment. Several days ago, however, she suddenly began to wheeze, and yesterday her worsening condition forced her to take the bus to SFGH for help.

When we enter Mrs. Papandreo's room there is no doubt she has severe asthma. Her anxious eyes alone tell us she is suffering. We can hear her wheezing from the foot of her bed. Every cycle of the ventilator produces a loud, high-pitched resonating whistle that gradually fades as her lungs fill with air, but then returns almost as loudly with each exhalation. We increase her sedation to give her a rest, and settle in for a lengthy and arduous course in trying to get her extubated.

Alexandra Papandreo came to us with what is called "adult-onset asthma," which is always a troubling diagnosis. "Classic" asthma usually begins in childhood and then takes one of two courses: children with mild involvement frequently outgrow their disease; in contrast, children with severe wheezing or chronic cough are apt to remain asthmatic throughout their lives. True asthma can certainly begin in adulthood, but it seems to me that Mrs. Papandreo's lung disease is not new and that her heavy cigarette smoking has caused slowly progressive chronic emphysema and bronchitis. These are chiefly responsible for her recent wheezing.

On this day alone we have three patients in the ICU with a component of asthma complicating severe chronic obstructive pulmonary disease, the fourth most common cause of death in the United States. From seeing all the harm cigarettes do, I have long been a fanatic antismoking crusader. A few years ago, people coming to dinner at our house would fidget miserably during the meal, then leave the table for a quick smoke outdoors. These fugitive absences are rare now because almost all our friends who smoked have quit.

Since his dangerously distended colon was decompressed, Francis Zohman has done well, though he has wheezed continuously during his thirty-six hours in the unit. I consider giving him more prednisone, but he is taking so much now that I am reluctant to raise the dose. His abdomen is less distended and tense. Because the danger of rupture has passed, I decide to transfer him. He is glad to leave and says, "Get me out of here, Doc. I'm scared of this place. Every time I come in, I get sick."

Howard McVicker's wife phoned me this morning with her concern about her husband's lack of improvement. I share it. He continues to resist our best efforts to identify and control any reversible elements of his disease. He keeps having asthma brought on by panic attacks despite steadily increasing intravenous doses of sedatives. As I had to tell her, lamely, all we can do is keep pushing his medications in the hopes that, with time and more drugs, his asthma will remit.

The decisive feature of asthma is that it is at least partially reversible. The air passages constrict in response to stimuli such as allergens, air pollutants, or even exercise, and the disturbance resolves as the airways dilate back to normal, sometimes spontaneously but often only in response to medications. We know that Mr. McVicker has severe chronic irreversible lung disease, but the fact that his wheezing and breathlessness come and go means he has an element of asthma too—and that, inherently, should be reversible. I have learned from Howard McVicker's clinic doctor, a colleague of mine on the faculty, that Mr. McVicker's physical activities had been restricted by breathlessness when he became too lively. Nevertheless, he had recently been going to the park every day to visit with his friends and was enjoying life greatly—until his asthma worsened, requiring this latest hospitalization. In theory, then, if we can control the complicating asthma, we should be able to get him back to the same pleasant life he delighted in before this attack began. The trouble is that we cannot identify the trigger for the episodes, and we are having much more than the usual struggle controlling the reversible element of his respiratory difficulties.

The last patient we see is Claudia Jonson. During the last day "the one-hoss shay" has not improved at all: the results of this morning's tests show that her uremia is worsening and that she has accumulated more fluid in her lungs. She will open her eyes when we shout her name, but she will not turn her eyes or head toward the origin of the sound. We do this repeatedly, and eye-opening is the maximum neurologic response we get, indicating greatly depressed brain function. There is no doubt now that she is thoroughly poisoned by her own blood

toxins and needs dialysis, which the nephrologists (kidney specialists) plan to
perform later in the day.

The impurities that accumulate in uremia are in many respects like a
large dose of sedative medications: they dull the mind and make it impossible to evaluate how well the brain is working. Thus, another reason
for dialyzing Ms. Jonson is to clear the uremia so that she can wake up
as much as possible. She seems to have suffered substantial brain damage, but in the presence of such severe kidney failure there is no way of
telling how much. Dialysis will help to sort it out.

A nice thing about this group of third-year residents is that they work
so well together, always helping one another. After we finish ward rounds
shortly after noon, Ella Andrews—who did not sleep at all last night and
must be exhausted after a hectic twenty-four hours on call followed by a
long morning of rounding—stays to help her buddies get Jaime Aguinaldo ready for the repeat endoscopy of his dilated blocked esophagus,
change Gertrude Davies's arterial cannula to avoid her broken arm, and
put a new cannula into Irwin Babcock to better monitor his shock from
who-knows-what. Ella's irrepressible good nature and enthusiasm are a
tremendous resource in the ICU and are contagious; she gives everyone
around her an emotional lift.

I too spend most of the afternoon in the ICU. About 2:30, as I am
making notes, I am relieved to see Alfredo Fiorelli wheeled back into
his room, returning from his prostate surgery in astonishingly good
condition.

DAY	
9	*Friday*

In 1964, Associate Justice Potter Stewart, unable to define obscenity in delivering his opinion of a case that had been heard before the Supreme Court, wound up with what has become one of the most widely quoted judicial pronouncements of all time: "but I know it when I see it." In a similar sense, with just a little information plus intuition, experienced ICU physicians "know" that a patient has pneumonia, gastrointestinal hemorrhage, or stroke when they see them. That is a valuable beginning, but it is not good enough: we must know more. Effective treatment requires knowledge of the *cause* of the condition. The more serious the problem, the more exigent the need for precision, especially in patients who have infections or are bleeding.

In the ICU, though, we rarely have time to make an exact diagnosis before starting therapy. We get what facts we can from the patient (or, because the patients are often unable to communicate, from friends or relatives and from old medical records); we perform a physical examination; and we check the results of rapidly available laboratory tests. From this information, we have to make an educated guess about the probable cause of the illness and begin empirical but life-saving treatment. Specimens are sent off to laboratories, and studies are ordered in hopes of confirming—later—the particular diagnosis we have chosen from among the candidates. In dangerously ill patients, like Irwin Babcock, the initial therapeutic barrage must be broad enough to cover even remote diagnostic possibilities. Jim Shotinger's patient last night was not as desperately sick, but he had to use the same "hope-we-got-it-covered" approach as a first-line intervention. There was no alternative if he didn't want her to get much worse.

■

Compared with Ella Andrews's frantic on call stint the day before, Jim has had a much calmer day. Only one new patient, Barbara Rivera, and she has been admitted to the ICU only two hours before we started ward rounds. Mrs. Rivera is a fifty-six-year-old divorcee who lives with her son and daughter-in-law; they brought her, over her objections, to the emergency department about 2:00 in the morning because her coughing and choking were keeping everyone in the house awake. She has mild pneumonia, ordinarily a condition that would be treated at home with easy-to-take oral antibiotics. But while getting dressed and preparing to leave the hospital, with her sleepy family restlessly waiting, she suddenly slumped over in her chair, turned blue, lost control of her bladder, and was unresponsive for about two minutes. So she was not sent home as planned but was admitted instead to the ICU. Her son's anxiety at going home without her was not relieved by his wife's pointing out they could finally get some sleep.

When we see Mrs. Rivera she is wide awake and totally responsive. Between coughs, she says, apologetically, "This is unbelievable! I didn't want to come here at all, and now I'm in intensive care. It was only a spell, so why don't you just send me home?" Although she seems to be doing well on the antibiotic Jim has chosen, I decide to keep her in the ICU until tomorrow, largely because of her "spell."

The decision to keep Barbara Rivera for observation is what is known in the institution as a "soft call," slightly more reason-based than a hunch. Betty Grambling, the head nurse in the surgical unit, disagrees with me.

"We don't need that woman in here," she argues. "She's not sick enough, and we need to open a bed." I defend my judgment by pointing out that Mrs. Rivera has been in the unit only a few hours, and it is too early to know if she is going to respond to the antibiotic we have given her. More compelling, we have no explanation whatsoever for her transient loss of consciousness in the emergency department.

Francis Zohman was not transferred out of the ICU yesterday as planned because his wheezing suddenly worsened and he started to complain about it. Additional cortisone was given intravenously, and he was held in the unit. Keeping him proved to be a wise decision, because he gradually worsened despite intensified treatment. About 5:00 this morning, he was no longer able to exhale enough carbon dioxide, which created an intolerable buildup of acid in his body. It was no longer safe to continue treating him in hopes that his asthma would soon mend. He had to be intubated right then, and he was.

Everything had been done to avoid intubating Francis Zohman. We wanted to avoid intubation because we knew, as we had been repeatedly reminded, by the examples of Truman Caughey and Howard McVicker, that once you put an endotracheal tube into someone with far-advanced chronic obstructive pulmonary disease it may have to stay in an insufferably long time and often becomes immensely difficult to take out. But we had to do it.

Next, we see Jaime Aguinaldo, the healthy-looking patient with the giant esophagus. Yesterday, the plan we invented during ward rounds was executed perfectly. The anesthesiologists had come to the unit and slipped an endotracheal tube into Mr. Aguinaldo's windpipe after giving him an anesthetic; then, while his lungs were protected from the entrance of liquids and he was asleep, a mini-

hose was passed through his mouth and throat into his esophagus, and a large amount of liquid blood, blood in clots, stringy residue from clots (fibrin), and barium were washed out by repeated rinses. Finally, he was ready to be reendoscoped. This time, it was possible to see that there was a one-inch tear in the lining membrane of his huge esophagus, which surely had been the cause of his bleeding. The endoscopist also found no cancer or other abnormality at the end of his esophagus or in his stomach; the mechanical obstruction was caused by unremitting spasms of the ring of muscle, the sphincter, that encircles the junction between the esophagus and stomach. Mr. Aguinaldo has a rare type of esophageal muscle disturbance called "achalasia." After the procedure it took about an hour for Mr. Aguinaldo to wake up sufficiently to be safely extubated.

Now, when we see him on ward rounds twenty hours later, everything is fine. He is in good spirits and wants to go home. It is too soon for that, so we try to reassure him by saying we will transfer him out of the ICU this afternoon for treatment of his correctable condition.

Achalasia, an uncommon disorder, occurs because the tubular layers of muscle in the wall of the esophagus do not function properly. There is both an absence of the rhythmic contractions, "peristalsis," that normally propel material through the esophagus into the stomach, and a failure of the sphincter at the junction where the esophagus joins the stomach, which is supposed to open and close like a shutter-valve, to relax and allow food and liquids to enter the stomach freely. Thus, swallowed material accumulates in the esophagus and forces its wall to gradually distend, sometimes to colossal dimensions.

Dr. Adrian Twist, one of our esteemed thoracic surgeons, wants to cut out Mr. Aguinaldo's entire esophagus and replace it by cutting loose part of his colon and bringing the freed portion up into the chest to provide a substitute swallowing tube, a horrendous operation. "No, no, no!" shouts the chief gastroenterologist, stamping his right foot thunderously with each "no." I am sure he is absolutely right, and as the physician in charge, I would never allow that kind of surgery. I can't help but admire, though, the way the gastroenterologist responds to this preposterous suggestion. The swallowing problems of achalasia, of which Mr. Aguinaldo has remarkably few, can usually be mitigated much more easily and safely: you can overpower the contracted ring of muscle by suddenly stretching it from within, using a pressure-actuated balloon. This is the treatment we plan to use first on him. Or you can inject the strong muscle relaxant botulinum (the same paralytic toxin that causes botulism, an often fatal kind of food poisoning) directly into the sphincter to overcome its spasm.[1]

Howard McVicker developed a fever at 6:00 A.M., despite the broad-coverage antibiotics he has been on for three days. He still has bursts of wild agitation accompanied by brisk increases in his heart rate and blood pressure. These episodes call for extra sedation, which explains his zombielike state this morning. His wife, terrified at his appearance, corners me; I tell her what's going on and add that we cannot cut back on the support provided by the ventilator until he wakes up more. Hearing this, his nurse, Jack Cramer, implores us not to reduce his sedatives very much. Since learning from the night nurse that Mr. McVicker almost pulled out his endotracheal tube, he is rightly concerned that it might happen again.

Irwin Babcock, the man who was admitted yesterday morning in deep shock shortly after injecting himself with a street mixture of methamphetamine, and who may also have a bloodstream infection complicating his HIV-induced immune suppression, is better than when we last saw him. He still requires an intravenous pressor to maintain his blood pressure, but we are pleased to hear that his output of urine has increased prodigiously without pharmacological nudging. He has eliminated over four quarts of the excess fluid he received yesterday in the throes of propping up his dwindling blood pressure.

Two big problems remain. First, Irwin Babcock continues to require medication to keep his blood pressure up, a sure sign of an ongoing serious problem. Second, we have no idea what is making him so sick. The cause is still a toss-up between a poison in the material with which he injected himself and septic shock, for which we are treating him. So far, we have been unable to find an obvious source of infection, and none of the many specimens we have collected and sent to the bacteriological laboratory has begun to grow a microorganism. Because we are working in total darkness, but our patient is getting better, I follow one of the golden rules of medicine—"when you are on a winning course, stay there." We leave everything we are doing exactly the same.

Alexandra Papandreo has many of the same formidable problems as Howard McVicker; both are susceptible to panic attacks, which bring on wheezing, rapid heart rate, and high blood pressure. These impromptu episodes are probably partly triggered by "ICU terror," a near-psychotic combination of drug-induced mania, frantic reflex signals to reject the endotracheal tube, and irrepressible fear of the ICU itself. When we examine her, Mrs. Papandreo is still wheezing loudly enough for us to hear without our stethoscopes. Nothing else has changed much either. Her failure to improve after thirty-six hours of the best treatment we have to offer is disappointing. We have no recourse except to press on with more of the same, and hope we aren't scaring her to death.

Next, we all move to the corner room to see Gertrude Davies, who was originally admitted to the ICU for surgical treatment of her fractured arm. After we saw her yesterday morning, she went to the x-ray department for a CT examination to look for blood in her abdomen, something that would explain her steadily declining hematocrit. She did not tolerate either the trip or the proce-

dure well, and she required extra intravenous fluids and two blood transfusions to reinforce her blood pressure, which kept dropping. Sometimes people near death are so fragile that merely moving them out of the ICU is dangerous. Much of the liquid she has received the last few days has leaked out of her blood-stream, which makes her face and skin puffy and waterlogs her lungs. She de-pends on the ventilator to give her weakened respiratory muscles a boost.

We have lots to remedy. We begin by trying to cut back on the intravenous fluids she is getting and by giving her a small dose of a diuretic to prod her kid-neys into producing more urine. We will also check to see if she can breathe without any help from the machine. We do not change the several antibiotics she was started on because her sites of infection appear to be coming under control. No one has seen her husband. Is he occupied in their dry-cleaning business, or has he abandoned her? Her social worker is not around to ask.

To finish up the morning's ward rounds, we go back upstairs to see the remain-ing two patients. The first is Claudia Jonson, who was dialyzed with good re-sults yesterday. The nurse-technician removed more than three quarts of extra fluid from her body. Now that her lungs are better, we decide to push aggres-sively forward with efforts to get her to breathe on her own. We still have to solve the major clinical riddle of how much brain injury she sustained on the several occasions when her blood pressure collapsed. She needs more dialysis, and we'll do it again today.

It was only yesterday morning when Alfredo Fiorelli went to the operating room for surgical drainage of his prostatic abscesses. Today he is much better. While we are examining him, Bart Reston, the urology resident, shows up to crow. I bite my tongue and thank him for his good work. He leaves convinced he saved Mr. Fiorelli's life. The operation certainly helped. A second, more sensitive, ul-

trasonographic study of Mr. Fiorelli's heart again shows that his widespread infection has spared his heart valves. He is lucky. Now he can be transferred to one of the medical wards.

The pus from Alfredo Fiorelli's prostate gland was overflowing with *Staphylococcus aureus*. This shows the importance of emptying pus pockets wherever they collect, and explains why the urologists were so eager to drain Mr. Fiorelli's abscesses. After three days of high-dose intravenous treatment with a potent synthetic penicillin, the bacteria were not only alive but thriving in their sequestered stockpiles. Antibiotics alone are often not enough.

TGIF, but no "Liver Rounds" today. Friday used to be the day of a regular celebration, called Liver Rounds, at SFGH and other teaching institutions. "Liver" implies that alcohol, with its medical connection with liver disease, will be served. The euphemism was useful because notices could be posted around the medical service reminding the housestaff and faculty where and when to show up; "Liver Rounds" created the impression among patients and their visitors that some sort of educational activity, not a drinking session, was being held. Patients, quite reasonably, do not like to think of their doctors carousing on duty—or ever, I sometimes think. Liver Rounds never was a place for serious drinking, only a beer or glass of wine at most, and the residents on call drank only cokes or soda. But the jolly events were a good occasion at the beginning of the weekend for housestaff and faculty to gossip and learn about each other.

Liver Rounds at the three University of California San Francisco hospitals have petered out, however. At SFGH the demise began a few years ago when a switch was made from beer and pretzels every Friday to supposedly more salubrious ice cream and chocolate chip cookies every once in a while. The prevailing theory for the expiration of Liver Rounds is sexist: it holds that the ritual faded when the predominantly male housestaff, who were accustomed to sitting around drinking beer together, shifted to a predominantly female housestaff, who had better things to do. Although to me it is still welcome, today's TGIF celebration beer will be drunk only when I get home, and with just my cat Walter to talk to.

Another weekend is starting, which means that most of the housestaff I meet will be wearing Robin Hood–green scrub suits, a loose-fitting blouse and baggy trousers originally designed to be worn only in the operating rooms but now worn by all medical residents and students when they are on call. It is easy to tell residents who are finishing a night on duty, not only from their sleep-seeking eyes but because their scrub suits are rumpled and sometimes spattered with blood or vomit. On-coming residents are clad in the same uniforms, but pristine and occasionally even ironed. Most of the scrub suits in evidence are "borrowed" from our operating room, although kept at home and washed by the owner. Occasionally, I see scrubs of other colors, liberated from other hospitals: blue ones labeled "UC Medical Center: Never to leave hospital" are most common; more rare is a gray trophy with "MGH-Boston" (Massachusetts General Hospital), a proud emblem of having gone to medical school at Harvard. Today, as on most weekends, green is everywhere because nearly all the housestaff are either post-call or starting call; the usual street-clothed crowd has the day off.

Today, though, it is hard to tell from appearances which of our two residents is coming on and which is going off duty. Ian Trent-Johnson has muddled my perceptions by taking a shower and putting on a fresh pair of scrubs minutes before rounds; not only that, he has shaved. He has had a hectic twenty-four hours, including the admission of five new patients and difficulties with the seven holdovers. He knows it is going to be a long morning, and he says, "I just needed to wash and clean up." After we finish our rounds with Ella Andrews, who is just arriving, he can change into his jeans and take off until Monday.

Because all the regular ICU beds are filled, the last of our newly admitted patients has to be cared for in the "PAR," the postoperative recovery room. We have to find another bed for him soon because the nurses there have their hands full caring for patients waking up from operations. Our posse takes the special elevator whose back doors open onto a warren of operating rooms. We go to see Luigi Califiano, a forty-six-year-old gay intravenous drug abuser known to be HIV-positive. Eighteen months ago his CD4+ T-cell count fell to $114/\mu l$, meaning he has AIDS.

Last week, he ran out of the antibiotic he had been taking to prevent Pneumocystis carinii *and other infections, and a few days later he developed chills, a stentorian cough, left-sided pleurisy, and shortness of breath. When he came to SFGH late last night with pneumonia, he was started on three antibiotics, each with broad firepower to cover most of the many possible causes of his infection. Then he was given a small amount of morphine to relieve his chest pain, which had become unbearable. His blood pressure immediately fell and did not respond either to an antidote for morphine, as it should have, or to more intravenous fluids. He was admitted to our ICU service rather than to a medical ward.*

When we see him a few hours after all this happened, he is wide awake and conversing intelligently about what is going on: "My chest still hurts terribly, but don't give me any more morphine; that's mean shit." A quick look at his record tells me he is urinating frequently and copiously. The ability to think and urinate tells us that his blood pressure, though still low numerically, is doing its job perfectly well. It is ensuring adequate blood flow to the brain and kidneys and does not need our attention. I decide to transfer Mr. Califiano to a medical ward right away, much to the relief of the nursing supervisor, who has been hanging around to make sure we move him.

This was an easy one. Luigi Califiano has all the earmarks of acute infectious pneumonia and nothing to suggest pneumocystis. The cause is almost certainly bacterial, a common and important complication of HIV infection in all of its stages. The antibiotic he had been taking to prevent pneumocystis fights off other germs, including several causes of community-acquired pneumonia. Thus his pneumonia and need for hospitalization might have been prevented had he continued the prophylactic medication he was supposed to take. Like many drug users, Mr. Califiano was not good about keeping his clinic appointments and renewing his medicines.

We head upstairs to review Milton Trageer, a twenty-three-year-old man who has been brought to SFGH by ambulance after being found in his downtown hotel room deeply comatose, incontinent, and frigid to the touch—seemingly dead. We know from his record that he is an insulin-dependent diabetic, but that is all. When he arrived in the emergency department yesterday about noon, his temperature was 78.8° F., his blood pressure was unobtainable, and his breathing was imperceptible. No pulse could be felt anywhere, and his pupils were dilated and fixed; that is, they did not constrict when a bright light was flashed in his eyes, signifying deep brain depression. The only way we knew he was alive was by an electrocardiographic monitor that revealed a heart rate of twenty-four beats per minute.

He was immediately intubated, given warm oxygen and hot intravenous fluids to combat the hypothermia, and medications to raise his blood pressure. Because his blood sugar level was elevated, and he had other chemical abnormalities of incredibly out-of-control sugar diabetes, he was treated with intra-

venous insulin and fluids. Later, someone noticed he had a slightly scaling red-dish rash over his trunk and extremities.

This morning he is much improved. To live, he had to improve; there was simply no physiologic room for him to get worse. His temperature is normal, he no longer needs drugs to sustain his blood pressure, and his prodigious metabolic abnormalities are gradually correcting. I put on gloves to examine him because the resident in dermatology thought Mr. Trageer's rash might be due to sec-ondary syphilis, which at this stage is highly contagious. He is flailing around in bed but is still intubated, which makes it difficult to determine how awake he is. Review of his initial chest x-ray, the one taken yesterday afternoon and the film made just this morning show healthy lungs to begin with, then progres-sively worsening pulmonary edema. We cut back on his intravenous fluids, con-tinue the insulin, and try to see if he can breathe by himself.

Milton Trageer is a lucky man. By clinical criteria—the absence of pulse, blood pressure, and respiration, and the presence of dilated fixed pupils—he was dead on arrival at SFGH. Only the electrocardiographic monitor showed cardiac activity. This example illustrates how difficult it can be to determine if someone is dead when his or her body tempera-ture is extraordinarily low. It underscores the wisdom of the old rule, "never dead until warm and dead." Mr. Trageer had diabetic coma com-plicated by hypothermia, an unusual association but one that is de-scribed in medical journals. He survived because of his youth and su-perb treatment by physicians not much older than he. He continued to improve and was extubated less than an hour after we saw him on ward rounds. Soon afterward, the chief of dermatology saw Mr. Trageer and diagnosed his skin rash as pityriasis rosea, a common dermatitis that resembles secondary syphilis.

After he woke up fully, Mr. Trageer told us he had run out of insulin four days before his admission. "I was going to get some more," he said, and that was the last thing he remembered. Nearly dying did not con-vince him to take his insulin every day; he has already had two subse-quent admissions to SFGH for uncontrolled diabetes mellitus. These

episodes keep recurring despite serious discussions about the uncondi-
tional necessity of his using insulin every day.

Mr. Trageer is by no means the only person who fails to take his
medicine regularly. He is particularly illustrative of the perilous consequences because when he does not inject his insulin he rapidly develops
life-threatening diabetic coma. Yet he still does not use it. As many as
half of all people with serious chronic diseases, such as heart failure,
asthma, and high blood pressure, and even curable infections like tuberculosis—which requires treatment for six months—do not take their
medications as prescribed. Reasons patients give for their high rate of
abstention are that the medicines have a bad taste or unpleasant side
effects and are inconvenient to administer or too expensive. A common
mistake is for people to stop their medications prematurely, as soon as
they feel better. Other factors that contribute are alcoholism, drug
abuse, homelessness, and mental illness; high levels of education and in-
come, however, do not guarantee that people will take their medications. How to ensure compliance with treatment, by whatever means—
teaching, browbeating, or inducements—remains one of the biggest
problems facing contemporary medicine.

*Next we see Herman Haagsman, an eighty-two-year-old man who was
brought in by ambulance last night. A member of one of the San Francisco Bay
Area's new prepaid health plans, he had been treated with x-ray therapy for
throat cancer in one of their facilities six months ago. We were unable to obtain
details about this when we telephoned because their record room was closed
for the weekend. He was admitted for pneumonia with respiratory distress and
is already much better. He smiles, shakes my hand, and in his raucous, rasp-
ing voice says, "My breathing is tremendously improved." He has radiation-
induced brownish-red changes in the skin over his upper neck and jaw, and
signs of pneumonia over his right lung. Although his new chest x-ray is a little
worse, clinically he is responding well.*

Later that day, Herman Haagsman was transferred from our ICU to an ICU in the hospital owned by his group insurance provider. We were sure he had pneumonia, but we never learned why he became so phenomenally breathless the night of admission, or if throat cancer or its treatment was contributing to the problem. Judging from his discordant voice, I guessed that he must have a serious mechanical impairment in that region. Writing this now reinforces the frustration I felt at the time: after we had invested effort and resources and had developed an emotional stake in the outcome, Mr. Haagsman simply disappeared, without any follow-up whatsoever. Doctors used to keep in touch about patients, but the proliferation of Health Maintenance Organizations, the anchor of contemporary American medicine, in which time is money, has practically eliminated this.

We go down to the fourth floor to see a sixtyish man who has not yet been identified. Although probably Chinese, he is known as John Doe. He was brought to the hospital thirty-six hours ago, after being found by the police lying bloody and battered on the sidewalk. His nose was bleeding, and the right side of his face was swollen and bruised. At first he was agitated and combative. He tried to fight off and escape from the officers, who finally arrested him and brought him to the hospital in handcuffs. Soon after he arrived in the emergency department, he lapsed into a coma.

Because of the possibility of trauma to his brain, the neurosurgeons were called; he was intubated and given a drug that paralyzed every muscle in his body so that a reliable CT scan of his head could be obtained. It showed no abnormalities. After nearly a full day of observation, his doctors concluded that he did not have a neurosurgical condition, and they transferred him to the medicine service. Because John Doe had been arrested and was in police custody, an officer from the Sheriff's Department has been at his side constantly—even while paralyzed inside the CT scanner or comatose in the surgical ICU, which is where we find him.

When we descend on him he is waking up, but his heart rate and blood pressure go up and down as he thrashes around, shaking the bed by the four canvas straps that restrain his arms and legs. The uniformed officer guarding him is in a chair at the bedside impassively reading the morning newspaper. The butt of a revolver in a holster at his right hip and a huge billy club suspended at his left hip make his sitting awkward. John Doe has shaken off the sheet covering the lower half of his body, displaying the plastic catheter emerging from his shrunken penis. His terrified eyes, peering out from their swollen black and blue surroundings, follow me as I listen to his heart and lungs. He tries to squirm out of the way when I poke his abdomen and press the skin over his ankle bones to find out if his feet are swollen. He looks at me beseechingly: why are you doing this to my helpless body? What is going on? His panic is so evident, I turn, smile warmly, and say, "You're in the hospital, San Francisco General Hospital, and now you're much better. Everything is on schedule, and we should be able to take that tube out soon. We'll see if it's safe right now."

"I'm sure he can't understand you," says Jack Cramer, Mr. Doe's nurse. "I've been talking to him since he started to wake up, but I haven't made contact. I don't think he speaks English."

"That's probably it," I agree, "so please get an interpreter up here right away. Imagine what it must be like to wake up in an ICU in a foreign country, face all battered, tied down, everyone around you speaking gibberish, and you can't utter a word because someone has shoved a tube down your throat. I travel a lot and have nightmares that this might happen to me. He looks Chinese, so let's start with that."

"He is Chinese, and I'll tell him now," volunteers a tall lanky young man, who steps forward wearing a starched white coat with a badge that introduces him as a UCSF medical student, Andrew Wu. And he does, after switching to a tonal voice with syllables going up and down, and the last one drawn out like the reverberation of a temple drum.

None of us bystanders has the faintest notion what Andrew Wu is saying, but the effect on John Doe is instantaneous. He stops struggling, smiles hugely, and his eyes begin to sparkle. It is not easy to smile with an endotracheal tube protruding from your mouth, especially when it is accompanied by a bulky plas-

tic mouthpiece, which we insert to prevent the patient from champing down and biting the tube. Mr. Doe manages anyway.

I ask Andrew what he has said. "I only repeated what you tried to tell him, but he couldn't have understood much. I spoke to him in Mandarin, which isn't his dialect. I suppose he speaks Cantonese, practically a different language."

"He understood enough," I comment. "The effect was miraculous. You get high marks for the day." Andrew's smile is almost as gigantic as John Doe's.

At the outset, there was good reason to suspect that John Doe's brain was injured when he was beaten up, but the neurosurgeons found no damage. Given his initial agitated clinical state and his subsequent coma, I concluded he had probably overdosed on something, most likely cocaine, an impression that was confirmed later in the day when the results came back of the chemical search of his urine for toxic substances. He was quickly extubated, and shortly afterward one of his nephews arrived and identified the patient as Wei-chi Chiang, a recent immigrant from Guangzhou. After a three-day wait, his family had finally called the police. They were used to his long absences while he gambled at pic joe (a fast-moving game, played with short sticks, which is popular among Chinese men), and they knew he smoked heroin from time to time. They seemed surprised to learn, however, that he was also snorting cocaine. No charges were ever filed, and he walked out of the hospital the next day.

The last of the new patients, Jean-Claude Lebrun, thirty-eight years old, was diagnosed with AIDS nearly five years ago when he developed Pneumocystis carinii *pneumonia. Since then he has had fewer than the usual morbid complications of HIV-induced pulverization of his body's defenses. (This is actually common now in patients taking highly active anti-HIV treatment, but this was before these medications became available.) Three days ago, he was admitted to*

the AIDS ward at SFGH for worsening dry cough and breathlessness, and with
a chest x-ray in which both lungs were peppered with countless tiny nodular
densities. Everything was so characteristic of a recurrence of P. carinii *pneu-*
monia that he was immediately started on the best available combined anti-
biotic preparation for the disease and given prednisone. A few hours later, ex-
amination of a specimen of sputum, induced by the reliable fine-mist technique
we used to diagnose Hugh Martini (Day 5), proved that Pneumocystis para-
sites were definitely present. He held his own for two days but then, as Ian
Trent-Johnson wrote in his note, "he crashed," with a precipitous decline in ar-
terial blood oxygen, accompanied by a rise in carbon dioxide and formation of
acidosis. Mr. Lebrun was immediately intubated and transferred to the ICU.
Then, his blood pressure dropped and he was started on an intravenous pressor
medication. A blood transfusion was ordered.

As we go in to meet him, I summon a big smile and say, "Bonjour, Monsieur
Lebrun, comment ça va?"

His mystified expression is explained when Ian leans over, grinning, and
whispers, "He's American, not French."

It is hard to believe that Mr. Lebrun is only thirty-eight years old; he looks
ancient and decayed, with sunken eyes, scrawny limbs, and a ghostly pallor. His
lungs sound as though they are overflowing with secretions, and his chest x-ray
reveals considerable progression of his disease since admission.

There is no doubt about the diagnosis of *P. carinii* pneumonia, and
everything has been done flawlessly to treat it from the moment Jean-
Claude Lebrun entered the hospital. Like many of our AIDS patients,
he is uncommonly knowledgeable about HIV disease and knows exactly
where he stands in its continuum. He was intubated last night because
he told his doctors he "wanted to be," and he also wanted to be sup-
ported aggressively so long as there was a "reasonable chance for recovery." But he added that he did not want his life "needlessly prolonged."
I know from past experience that there is a small window of opportunity
in patients who have just developed respiratory failure from pneumo-

cystis. He was newly intubated and sedated, so I cannot discuss the matter with him, but after learning his wishes, I decide to write a "do not resuscitate" order. If his heart ceases beating, we will not try to restart it. Mr. Lebrun is already getting all we have to offer, and if his heart stops, his body is sending a message we should pay attention to. Restarting his heart with thumps or shocks might add a few hours or days to his life, but it will not change the final outcome. His mother and sister agree. There is nothing left for any of us to do but to wait and see if his body's survival skills will prevail.

The first of our old patients we see is cortisone-ravaged Francis Zohman, the patient with asthma and chronic lung disease we had to intubate yesterday morning during a precipitous attack of asthma. To make matters worse, at 11:00 P.M. more drama started when his blood pressure collapsed. When Ian Trent-Johnson examined Mr. Zohman's chest with his stethoscope, he could not hear the usual sounds of air entering and leaving the left lung. An emergency chest x-ray revealed that his entire left lung had shrunk in size and become opaque, indicating that it no longer contained air. This sometimes occurs when the endotracheal tube works its way beyond the windpipe into the main bronchial passage to the right lung. In doing so, it blocks entry of air to the left lung. But the x-ray showed that the tube was exactly where it ought to be, in the lower third of the windpipe. Ian made the correct diagnosis of a plug of mucus obstructing the central air passage to the left lung. He asked Mr. Zohman's nurse to suction him vigorously with a narrow plastic catheter that she passed into the bronchial tubes through the endotracheal tube. The respiratory therapist turned the patient first on one side and then on the other so that she could clap each side of his back with her hands, as in smacking the bottom of a catsup bottle, in an effort to dislodge the plug.

These maneuvers worked. ICU medicine is often no more sophisticated than this. His blood pressure jumped up to its previous level, and the oxygen defi-

ciency in his blood corrected. This morning he is the best I have seen him, though he still requires an endotracheal tube and a machine to breathe satisfactorily.

■

We then see Barbara Rivera, the fifty-six-year-old woman with pneumonia, who was admitted to the ICU after she lost consciousness in the emergency department. We had been tempted, and encouraged, to transfer her out of the unit yesterday morning after rounds. For mainly intuitive reasons, I elected to keep her a little longer to see how things unfolded—a prudent decision as it turned out. Yesterday afternoon her fever declined and she was feeling much better, but later in the evening she had another episode of turning blue and passing out, exactly like the "spell" she had in the emergency department.

This time, because her heart rate and level of oxygenation were being monitored by our instruments, we could tell exactly what happened. First of all, her oxygenation started to decrease, then her heart rate became perilously slow, and, moments later, she lost consciousness. Betch Minerva, her nurse, recognized what was going on and quickly passed a suction catheter into Mrs. Rivera's windpipe, which made her cough violently. A large quantity of thick, purulent secretions issued from her lungs, that Betch sucked out. Mrs. Rivera's heartbeat abruptly quickened, her oxygenation leapt, and she awakened. This told us that the muscles she uses for coughing or the reflexes that actuate them have become weary from days of overwork. No longer can they do their job unless provoked by suctioning. Now that we know what is going on, it is safe to transfer her to the intermediate care unit, where skilled nurses and respiratory therapists can help Mrs. Rivera get rid of her excess secretions by suctioning, as Betch was forced to do, or by physical therapy, as was done to Francis Zohman, if she cannot do it by herself.

Without coughing, people with pneumonia can drown in their own juices. They need to cough repeatedly and forcefully to empty their airways of the purulent secretions produced deep within infected lungs.

When the act of coughing is weakened by muscle disease or debility, or the signals that provoke cough are depressed by alcohol or drugs, sputum accumulates in the air passages. If not removed, it obstructs the delivery of incoming fresh air to parts of the lungs, which impairs the oxygenation of blood. When severe, lack of oxygen slows the heart and ultimately depresses the brain, as we saw with Barbara Rivera. After her transfer, she did well and left SFGH five days later to finish her treatment at home.

We move on to the room of Claudia Jonson, our endearing patient with depressing medical problems, who has depended on dialysis to control her kidney failure and a ventilator to assist her breathing. After we saw her on ward rounds yesterday, she was dialyzed for the second time; again, more than three quarts of excess fluid were removed. As expected, today's blood tests show that her uremia is better, and the morning's chest x-ray reveals that her pulmonary edema is nearly gone. Her neurologic examination, however, has not changed: automatonlike, she opens her eyes every time I shout her name, but that is all the response I can provoke.

Since her admission to the ICU we have made a little headway in cutting back on her need for machine-supported breathing. We'll continue to wean her during the weekend. We also request a CT scan of her head, using a special iodine-containing dye to spotlight any anatomic abnormalities of her brain. The contrast material can be toxic to the kidneys, but we have to take that risk, and she is already being dialyzed. The scan is set for Monday.

Howard McVicker, who has been with us now sixteen days, has had a quiet twenty-four hours. The fever that worried us yesterday morning has disappeared. Even better is the news that the medications we started him on yester-

day have helped. He has been calmer than usual, and when we examine him, he is less wild-eyed and frightened looking. But we cannot tell if he is still psychotic since it is impossible to communicate with him. Because his weight has increased, raising the possibility that his recent wheezing and poor oxygenation are related to occult pulmonary edema from excess fluids, I tell his nurse to give him a diuretic to rid his lungs of any extra water that might have accumulated there. This kind of physiological fine-tuning can sometimes produce striking benefits, but you never know until you try.

The HIV-infected patient, Irwin Babcock, who was admitted to the ICU in shock two days ago, still requires intravenous pressor medications to counteract the persistent tendency of his blood pressure to fall. We still do not know whether he injected a contaminating poison along with the methamphetamine just before he became so violently ill, or whether he was, and is, seriously infected.

The dry-cleaner owner with a fractured arm and malnutrition, Gertrude Davies, is no better this morning, and her chest x-ray is a little worse. Yesterday she had a trial off the breathing machine to see if she could breathe by herself. After only two hours she tired and had to be reconnected again. We decide to try another weaning technique, one in which we withdraw support gradually, as tolerated, until she breathes completely on her own.

Our third and last asthmatic to be seen this morning, Alexandra Papandreo, is not wheezing as loudly as she has before, which we interpret as slight progress. Her hematocrit, however, has continued to decrease. Soon she'll need a blood transfusion.

Ian, Ella, and I return to the ICU from the x-ray department this morning later than usual. Neurologists are scarce on weekends, but we had to find one to review Milton Trageer's and John Doe's CT scans. As we walk in, we are greeted by bright-eyed Pauline Victoria who fixes us with her gaze and says, "Oh, what a shame; you just missed Mr. Palacio and Roxy, Constancia Noe's father and sister. They came in to thank everybody, and they asked especially about all of you. And they brought us a big box of candy, over on the counter, but you better hurry, it's going fast." The contents had nearly disappeared: by the time we got to it, both layers had been rifled and my favorites, chocolate-covered nuts, were gone.

DAY	
11	*Sunday*

We worry a lot about oxygen in the ICU. Without oxygen to the brain, a person becomes unconscious in about thirty seconds and is dead a few minutes later. Oxygen is needed for the heart to beat, for the liver to synthesize proteins, for the kidneys to manufacture urine, for all cells to live and function. Oxygen keeps the "fires of life" burning by furnishing metabolic fuel for all creatures in the animal kingdom, from microscopic amoebas to colossal blue whales. Nature has designed highly refined pathways to transfer oxygen from the surrounding water or air to the chemical furnaces deep within each cell where oxygen is consumed in the metabolic processes that generate energy.

In humans, as in other higher animals, the first step along the oxygen pathway is breathing, the process that brings oxygen-containing fresh air into the microscopic air sacs of the lungs. Oxygen molecules diffuse across the delicate membranes that line these sacs and their adjacent capillaries, and the molecules penetrate the interior of circulating red blood cells where oxygen combines chemically with a protein carrier called "hemoglobin." The presence of normal amounts of hemoglobin in the bloodstream enables the lungs to deliver to the tissues sixty times more oxygen than blood without it. The heart pumps oxygen-rich blood through the branching system of arteries and capillaries into every organ. At the end of their journey, oxygen molecules leave their hemoglobin carrier, diffuse out of the capillaries and across the external membranes of neighboring cells, and enter the subcellular elements, "mitochondria," where oxygen is instantly burned in a miniature explosion that creates life-giving energy.

Oxygen must be constantly fed into this intricate supply line and through its hungry tributaries, or disaster strikes quickly. That is why we constantly check with arterial blood studies and oximeters to ensure that our ICU patients are getting enough. Today, as is often the case, each of our nine patients is breathing extra oxygen; some need it more than others, but it adds an element of safety to everyone.

Our only new patient, Eduardo Quetzel, a thirty-eight-year-old unemployed construction worker, was summoned from his hotel to SFGH yesterday because the results of laboratory studies obtained the day before in the outpatient department showed that he probably had an alarming infection in his abdominal cavity. His illness began six months ago with progressive abdominal swelling from fluid (ascites) caused by severe alcoholic liver disease; the fluid disappeared after he decreased his intake of salt and started taking diuretic pills. Recently, the swelling began to recur, this time accompanied by pain. Two days ago, Mr. Quetzel went back to the clinic, where his doctor withdrew some of the fluid into a syringe and sent the specimen to the laboratory. The material contained many pus cells, signs of a grave infection called "spontaneous bacterial peritonitis." Yesterday, as soon as his clinic doctor received this ominous report, she telephoned the manager at Mr. Quetzel's hotel, who relayed the message that he should return to SFGH at once. He was feeling even worse than he had the day before, so he came to the hospital and was admitted to a medical ward right away.

At 5:00 this morning, just three hours before we started rounds, the night nurse found him unconscious and barely breathing. He was intubated forthwith and transferred to us. When we examine him, he is comatose, his jaundice has deepened to bright canary yellow, his belly and legs are colossally bloated, and he is in shock. His kidneys have made almost no urine, and their failure to function has contributed to a rise in the concentration of potassium in his blood to a level that threatens to stop his heart. We can lower his potassium level with drugs, but that would only be temporizing. To keep him alive longer requires dialysis, a difficult and dangerous procedure for someone in shock. The kidney specialists are reluctant to start; they confirm our impression that Mr. Quetzel has "hepatorenal syndrome," kidney failure secondary to liver failure, a combination that is nearly always fatal.

Although the deterioration first of Eduardo Quetzel's liver and now of his kidneys has been swifter than usual, there is nothing we can do about it, so we decide not to try. He is dying because he does not have enough functioning liver cells to carry out the liver's many metabolic tasks. Because his decline has been so unforeseen and rapid, his mother and girlfriend cannot believe, let alone accept, the idea that his death is near. "He should have stayed home," his pretty, much younger girlfriend keeps saying.

After we finish rounds, Jim Shotinger goes back to Mr. Quetzel's room to explain to them the hopelessness of the situation and the imminence of his demise. "No, no, it can't be true; he's stopped drinking," his girlfriend cries. "Eddy is too young. He's been sick only two days." His mother doesn't say a word as she sits by her son's side clutching his saffron-colored, puffy arm.

After lunch, Jim goes back and talks to them again. At 3:00 P.M., he notes in the chart, "They are beginning to understand." Less than an hour later, Mr. Quetzel is dead. His mother and girlfriend remain by his corpse, totally bewildered, unable to comprehend their loss.

Presiding over death is never easy. Even when we can do nothing for the patient, as with Eduardo Quetzel, we do what we can for the family. The kind of catastrophic illness we encounter in the ICU is often sudden, sometimes completely without warning, and leads to unimaginable despair in the unprepared family. When possible—for example with a young, formerly robust person who is decimated in seconds by a massive brain hemorrhage and comes in dying—I try to keep the patient alive an extra day, occasionally two, for the purpose of allowing the family to internalize the fact that the death cannot be avoided, and to give others time to travel to San Francisco to say good-bye. Not everyone would agree with my using the ICU this way, especially whoever is paying the bill.

After two days on the medical ward, Alfredo Fiorelli, the methamphetamine abuser we treated for more than four days for widespread staphylococcal infection and shock, was sent back to the ICU last night. His prostatic abscesses had been successfully drained, but he had other surprises in his body waiting to announce themselves. Yesterday morning, he started to vomit dark blood, and his hematocrit began to fall. After he arrived we gave him two blood transfusions. A fiberoptic endoscopy revealed an active duodenal ulcer. By the time we see him on rounds this morning, his condition has restabilized, and there is no further clinical or laboratory evidence of bleeding. We decide to transfer him back to the ward he came from with antibiotics and antacids to heal his ulcer.

As Alfredo Fiorelli is discovering, intravenous drug abuse is a hazardous pastime. Users have no way of knowing exactly how much or even what they are injecting into their bloodstream. Street drugs of uncertain origin are diluted with other substances, some toxic themselves. Overdosage is undoubtedly the most common complication and may be fatal. Another serious hazard is the transmission of infection—especially HIV, hepatitis, and bacteria—by contaminated syringes and needles. All our medical housestaff know what to do for a "shooter with a fever": draw two blood cultures, look for a source of infection, and start antibiotics, which must include coverage of *Staphylococci*, probably the most common of the likely germs. The problem is not solved simply by making a diagnosis and starting treatment; drug abusers are notoriously bad at complying with therapy. Even in the hospital, addicts cunningly conspire to inject themselves with heroin, cocaine, or other illicit drugs. The intravenous drips inserted for therapeutic reasons provide convenient access. We have even had deaths from overdosage in the hospital.

After Mr. Fiorelli's second transfer from the ICU to the ward, his severe staphylococcal infection slowly responded to treatment with intravenous antibiotics. Yet another abscess surfaced, this time next to his anus, and this also required drainage by surgeons. After sixteen days of treatment, he wanted to leave the hospital in spite of his doctors' pleas to stay for the entire course of twenty-eight days of intravenous therapy. He remained implacable and signed himself out of the hospital "against medical advice." He left SFGH with a supply of oral antibiotics for a hotel room that had been booked for him, where he was to be seen by a visiting nurse. He was also given an appointment in the Infectious Disease Clinic that he did not keep.

Leaving the hospital against medical advice is common practice among drug addicts and usually terminates vital therapy. We do not know exactly what happened to Mr. Fiorelli because he was never seen again. Unless he took the antibiotics he left the hospital with, there is a good chance that his infection recurred and killed him.

I know drug abusers are human beings, each with a personal tragedy that deserves sympathy, which I try to provide. As a group, though, addicts are difficult and frustrating patients. They construct medical histories that are full of misinformation and falsehoods; they will say almost anything, and creatively malinger, to get sedatives and narcotics. Addicts rarely listen to advice. They sign themselves out of the hospital all the time, and fail to return for follow-up visits. Alfredo Fiorelli is a typical example. Not unexpectedly, this atmosphere of constant deceit and its corollary deep mistrust among physicians—residents and attending physicians alike—retards diagnosis and treatment of addicts when they really do become sick.

Claudia Jonson, our transvestite who requires dialysis and machine-assisted breathing, has not changed. She continues to open her eyes to noisy stimuli but doesn't turn her head or make any purposeful movements. This morning's chest x-ray shows that her pulmonary edema is returning, which is to be expected because she has not been dialyzed for two days. We decide not to change the ventilator settings until she returns from the x-ray department later today after having the CT scan.

Irwin Babcock, the HIV-infected patient whose blood pressure collapsed an hour after he injected himself with methamphetamine, is doing fine at last. None of the many specimens we submitted to the bacteriology laboratory has revealed a causative germ. Because Mr. Babcock no longer needs ICU ministrations, we will send him to one of the medical wards.

Although we were very curious and tried hard to find out, we never learned what almost killed Irwin Babcock. I suspect that the "dirty crank" he injected contained a deadly contaminant. He remained hospitalized while receiving intravenous antibiotics for seven days and then was sent home to take antibiotics by mouth for another seven days. He refused all efforts at counseling or drug rehabilitation, but he did agree to go to one of our affiliated clinics for a follow-up visit and future care of his HIV infection, which he will surely need.

The recently available form of triple therapy for HIV infection is highly effective but quite costly ($10,000 to $12,000 a year). Most important, it has to be taken according to a strict regimen that is not easy to follow. Addicts, like Mr. Babcock, cannot be relied on to take any drugs other than their favorite illicit ones. For this reason, some have argued that addicts should not receive the new antiviral combinations if they become HIV-infected. Not only would this save money, it would minimize the risk of the virus's becoming resistant to the medications owing to irregular treatment. At SFGH the decision to treat drug abusers for HIV infection is individualized and is based on criteria such as whether or not they are in a rehabilitation program, return for follow-up visits, and have support from family or friends. We recognize that transmission of drug-resistant strains of HIV poses a real threat for the future.

We hear about Gertrude Davies, the patient with a fractured arm who needs machine-assisted breathing. Her diminutive nurse, Carol Ceruti, immaculate in her starched white uniform, reports that Mrs. Davies is no longer febrile and needs less suctioning than before to free her lungs of phlegm, a turn for the better that correlates with improvement in her chest x-ray. We decide to take advantage of this gain by accelerating the weaning schedule we launched yesterday. The skin over her buttocks is beginning to wear through and ulcerate, and her abdominal wound does not look good either. We conclude that, on balance, she is marginally improved.

Next we go to see Jean-Claude Lebrun, the patient with AIDS, who yesterday seemed to be dying from Pneumocystis carinii *pneumonia, and for whom I had written a "do not resuscitate" order. Because the first blood transfusion he received in the morning appeared to shore up his blood pressure, he was given a second and finally a third unit of blood, after which the pressor medications were no longer needed. His new chest x-ray is tremendously improved. There is only one explanation for this kind of rapid and spectacular clearing of someone's lungs: mobilization of pulmonary edema fluid. But there is no obvious reason why Mr. Lebrun's lungs should have wrung themselves out, and the three units of blood we gave him should have been counterproductive to this effect. We decide to augment this spontaneous but fortuitous physiological drying up by giving him a diuretic, but we will have to keep a keen eye on his blood pressure to ensure that it does not fall again as we deliberately deplete his body of fluids.*

Among our three intubated asthmatics with different types and degrees of chronic obstructive pulmonary disease, the first patient we see this morning is the newest one, Alexandra Papandreo, who should be getting better faster than she is. Ever since admission four days ago, her agitation-linked asthma has continued to wax and wane; this morning, we can hear it loudly waxing when we enter her room. The sole glimmer of hope is the fact that these intermittent setbacks seem to be less frequent than before. Yesterday, during a respite, she breathed without assistance from the machine for nearly four hours. We leave orders with the respiratory therapist to wait until the present attack subsides, and then to see if Mrs. Papandreo can breathe by herself again.

The second of these three asthmatics is puffy-faced Francis Zohman, the patient who came to the ICU five days ago when his colon was on the verge of rupturing. As that was improving, his asthma worsened to the point where he had to be intubated. When we examine him he is discouraged and depressed by his long hospitalization and failure to get better. Usually he smiles and welcomes our arrival; today he is withdrawn and morose. The endotracheal tube prevents him from conversing with us, but he is undoubtedly glum. The extra cortisone-type medications we have had to give him have worsened his already frightful-looking acne. Maybe this depresses him.

"How's it going, Mr. Zohman?" I ask, adding an affectionate pat on his shoulder. "They tell me everything's holding its own or mending." (If the truth

be known, much more of the former than the latter.) But he keeps his head turned away and spurns my efforts to cheer him up.

Last, we hear about Howard McVicker, who has developed a sustained fever since we saw him yesterday. His white blood cell count has risen, which reinforces the notion that he has an active process, probably an infection, somewhere in his body. But where? Two days ago Mr. McVicker's temperature jumped abnormally. It promptly subsided, and so we ignored it. This time we cannot.

The onset of fever is a tip-off that something, nearly always undesirable, is happening. Because a multitude of causes may increase a patient's temperature in the ICU, many things have to be done to unmask its source. The usual cause of fever is infection, so we check out and submit material for bacterial culture from the usual places where infection occurs: the lungs (sputum), kidneys (urine), indwelling vascular catheters (blood). And we do a thorough physical examination for clues: tenderness, swelling, or redness. Medications are reviewed for likely causes of allergic reactions—all drugs are potentially culpable, some more than others. If nothing turns up, we obtain a CT of the abdomen to look for an abscess or other occult source. Somewhere along this continuum, depending on how sick the patient is, antibiotics with an extended spectrum of activity are begun. Fever cannot be overlooked, but deciphering its cause can be time-consuming, costly, and frustrating—for patients and doctors alike.

We finish ward rounds and x-ray rounds on schedule at 10:30 A.M., and I complete my notes by 12:30 P.M. I have already lined up a tennis game later in the afternoon, so the sensible thing to do is to have lunch and work a bit in the hospital, as I did yesterday, before heading for my club in Berkeley. Today, though, I feel saturated with SFGH and need a break. Besides, I am feeling guilty about Walter, who is not getting his usual amount of attention because my wife is still in France doing research for a new book, and I am at the hospital all the time. I always let Walter out for a walk in the early morning before I leave home, and again in the evening when I return, but he prefers to check out his territory several times during the day. So I go home, and after Walter makes sure that no cats have moved into the block since his morning inspection, he joins me for a bite of the tuna sandwich I have fixed for lunch. Just then the telephone rings.

It is Jim Shotinger calling about a patient he is seeing in our AIDS ward. The man has been in the hospital a week for his third episode of *P. carinii* pneumonia, and he is not doing well. Two days ago his left lung collapsed from an internal rupture, and a large tube had to be inserted to keep the lung expanded. The tube is leaking air, and the patient's oxygenation is worsening. Should he be intubated and moved to the ICU? I do not say "definitely not," but I do my best to discourage it. At SFGH, patients with *P. carinii* pneumonia who require intubation for respiratory failure have a mortality rate of seventy-six percent. The presence of a collapsed lung, chest tube, and large airleak increases the likelihood of mortality to well over ninety percent. This is the patient's third episode of the disease, and he has not responded to a week of treatment, adverse features that raise the mortality even higher — close to one hundred percent. There is, perhaps, the slimmest of chances that he can survive this episode, but to find out would mean risking a long period of torture. Dying in increments with a tube in your windpipe and another in your chest is infinitely miserable. Even if he pulled through, underneath it all is advanced AIDS, for which he has received our best treatment but has failed to respond. I ask Jim to convey this information to the patient and his family because the final decision is theirs, not mine. I cannot deny but would recommend, strongly, against intubation and transfer to the ICU.

The master diagnostician of the turn of the century made almost as good use of his sense of smell as of his sight. Tales are still told about the astute clinician, on his way into a crowded ward with his entourage, stopping and sniffing at the threshold, then saying, "There is someone with a lung abscess in here." All the students, knowing that such a patient had been admitted the night before, would marvel at this wizardry. Some lung abscesses really do stink, and even I can recognize them at the bedside, though seldom at the entrance to the ward, by their fetid smell. Distinguished physicians of yesteryear were also reputed to diagnose uremia and diabetic coma by their characteristic odors. Today's physicians get little practice at this because most patients with kidney failure are dialyzed long before they reek of uremic toxins. Although you can smell acetone on the breath of an out-of-control diabetic with ketoacidosis, it quickly disappears with insulin and intravenous fluids.

I have not found a highly tuned sense of smell to be an advantage in the ICU because the prevailing odors are nearly always fecal in origin and powerfully offensive. Regardless of good intentions, the stench of stool and knowledge of what you will find under the covers manifestly restricts the extent of your examination and physical contact with an incontinent patient, sometimes with disastrous consequences. I have never forgotten the episode of years ago, when I was a first-year resident working in the emergency department. A patient was brought in who was layered from scalp to heel with feces, old and new. Everyone stood at a distance. Even the hardiest old veterans would not get near him. Finally someone decreed he had to be bathed. Five minutes after being put in the tub, while soaking, he died.

Patients are mortified by "accidents" when they are conscious, but sometimes the urge to defecate can be too powerful to contain. Even normal peristalsis can soil the bed when patients are sedated and unable to control themselves. Without knowing who or why, when I walk into the ICU this morning, a familiar rank odor assails me: someone with a brisk gastrointestinal hemorrhage is stooling in bed.

"Another bleeder," says Jim Shotinger, using our terse ICU slang, as we greet each other at the nurses' station. The endoscopists are also assembling, but they have stationed their television monitor and equipment outside the patient's room. I have always thought that gastroenterologists would get used to the odors they encounter all day. No, they are no more eager than I am to enter that evil-smelling room. We keep them at bay while the first-year resident informs us about the patient.

Amos Younger is a fifty-two-year-old man with cirrhosis of the liver, chronic alcoholism, and active hepatitis C virus infection. He left his wife and children many years ago and, after drifting from one city to another, decided to stay in San Francisco. Like so many of our patients who subsist on welfare, small pensions, or social security, he now lives in a cheap hotel. Last night the manager telephoned 911 after he found Mr. Younger on the floor of his room, drenched in plum-colored stool.

This morning, his low hematocrit has not increased at all after the transfusion of six units of blood. He must still be bleeding, an assumption reinforced by the recovery of bright red blood through the tube in his stomach and by his intermittent episodes of malodorous maroon-colored diarrhea. Though conscious, he makes no effort to use the bedpan when an irresistible wave of peristalsis ejects another pint of blood from his rectum. When we examine him, we find all the signs of cirrhosis of the liver, plus pulmonary edema and a loud heart murmur. We roll our eyes sympathetically at his gowned, gloved, and masked nurse, who cannot change the sheets fast enough to keep him clean, and hastily leave the room so the endoscopists can do their work.

Although Amos Younger has bled a lot and is still bleeding, his problem is complicated by pulmonary edema from heart disease, which makes it more of a juggling act to keep replacing only the amount of blood he is losing and not to transfuse more than his crippled heart can accommodate. What we really need to know is where all the blood is coming from. That will focus our attack, and perhaps the endoscopists can do something locally to stop the hemorrhage. In addition, Mr. Younger has passed our arbitrary clinical threshold of six units of blood, hence increasing the likelihood that he will need an operation to control the bleeding. No definitive decisions are possible, however, until a diagnosis of what is causing the bleeding can be established by endoscopy.

Claudia Jonson went to the x-ray department for the CT study of her head yesterday afternoon. Like many sick patients who cannot follow commands, she had to be sedated to prevent her from moving while the films were taken. The medications caused a transient drop in her blood pressure, but her condition stabilized quickly, and the study was completed satisfactorily.

We review the CT films with an expert neuroradiologist, who points out the considerable shrinkage of Ms. Jonson's brain but not much else. In response to my pointed questions the radiologist insists there is no evidence—not even a hint—of the characteristic abnormalities that can occur when the brain suffers from lack of oxygen. Maybe her brain is normal.

Maybe, though, it has been damaged. If the CT examination had un-covered destruction within the brain, we could be sure it had occurred. Because the technique is not sensitive enough to detect subtle but grave injury, a negative examination does not rule out the possibility that Claudia Jonson has sustained substantial brain damage. Magnetic reso-nance (MR) imaging of the brain is more sensitive than a CT study for discovering the abnormalities we are looking for, but, given the fragility she showed during yesterday's CT examination, an MR, which is more complicated for someone on a ventilator, is too risky. We have to depend on the neurologists' clinical examination, which means we must be more vigorous about dialysis.

Howard McVicker still has his unexplained fever. Yesterday, specimens of his blood, sputum, and urine were collected and sent to the bacteriology laboratory for culture, but we have not started new antibiotics. We have no clues to guide our selection, and I want to save the "big guns" for when they might be needed —if, for example, he becomes infected with one of the hospital's multiresistant superbugs.

This morning his belly is distended and tense from gas, and the gurgling sounds of normal peristaltic activity, which should be easily heard, are infrequent and barely audible. It is not much to go on, but his swollen quiet abdomen is our first lead to a source of fever and mischief. We start our investigation by order-ing x-rays of his belly and asking the surgeons to see him. His wife, who has re-arranged her work schedule to spend more time with him, mainly reading Danielle Steele because he cannot talk to her, senses our collective unease and asks if she should worry too. I reply, "Not just yet. Let's see what the x-rays turn up."

The former surgical patient with the fractured shoulder and slow-healing wounds, Gertrude Davies, is clearly better this morning. Yesterday, she so im-

pressed Jim Shotinger and the respiratory therapist that they twice tried her without any machine support at all, and she breathed well for two hours both times. When we see her on ward rounds, she is again breathing on her own and looks fine. She squeezes my hand wanly and squinches up her cheeks in a feeble attempt to smile. We decide that now is the time to let her breathe by herself for several more hours. If she continues to do as well, we will take the tube out. We still have not heard from her husband, or anyone else.

Unlike most asthmatics who are given large doses of cortisone-type drugs, Francis Zohman obstinately does not improve. He makes a little progress in one direction but loses ground in another. Meanwhile, the acne-producing side effects of prednisone are vividly apparent: his face continues to blossom. This morning we learn that yesterday he had two successful breathing trials of four hours each. This big step forward is more than offset by the news that on one occasion his oxygenation dropped alarmingly, though, as before, it responded to assiduous suctioning of his lungs. Moreover, Mr. Zohman's pulmonary secretions have been increasing in quantity and stickiness, which means more and more suctioning. This morning's chest x-ray is much worse; we find two large patchy densities, most likely zones of lung that are plugged by abundant tenacious phlegm. It's time to consider a tracheotomy, an idea that has been in the back of my mind for several days.

We do far fewer tracheotomies in ICU patients these days than we used to. This is because new soft plastic endotracheal tubes with low-pressure cuffs can be safely left in place for three or four weeks—plenty of time to treat whatever condition necessitated intubation in the first place. Nevertheless, we have made no headway with Francis Zohman, who has required three intubations this admission. And now we have to confront the new problem of complications from sticky phlegm. A tracheotomy facilitates the removal of secretions because it is easier to direct a suction catheter through a short tracheotomy cannula than through the much longer endotracheal tube. As we leave Mr. Zohman's room, I ask Ian to have the nose and throat surgeons see him.

◼

Alexandra Papandreo, the retired seamstress whose "adult-onset asthma" suddenly ballooned into acute respiratory failure about a week ago, has improved a little, but under difficult circumstances. She breathed without ventilator support for four hours yesterday, and everyone who saw her at the time said she looked "terrific." But without warning or discernible provocation an attack of asthma and wild agitation struck, requiring deep sedation and machine-assisted breathing. When we see her on rounds this morning she is breathing without the ventilator, but she is wheezing loudly and starting to get restless and have fits of coughing. Jack Cramer, her nurse today, is poised to sedate Mrs. Papandreo again and connect her back to the ventilator as soon as we finish our examination. I decide instead that Jack should give her a small amount of a rapidly acting tranquilizer to try to calm her a little, and to let her continue to breathe by herself as long as possible. We also leave an order to give her two units of blood because her hematocrit has fallen and she needs transfusion.

◼

We all go back to the fifth floor to see Jean-Claude Lebrun, our only remaining patient with AIDS, who continues to do astoundingly well. In response to a single low dose of a diuretic yesterday morning, he produced a large amount of urine. His blood pressure never flickered, and his oxygenation improved. All of this benefit is reflected in his new chest x-ray, which shows further resolution of the mixture of pneumocystis pneumonia and pulmonary edema. When we examine him he seems positively light-hearted and is able to take deep breaths and to cough, promising indicators of a successful trial to determine if he can breathe by himself.

We have come to the end of rounds and have not seen the patient with AIDS and *P. carinii* pneumonia that Jim Shotinger called me about at home yesterday afternoon. I ask him what happened. He tells me that after the patient, surrounded by his lover and family, heard the dire statistics that I provided over the phone, they all decided, without hesitation or disagreement, against transfer to the ICU for aggressive care. Jim adds that everyone, the patient included, seemed enormously relieved to know that his suffering would soon be over. Afterward, he continued to worsen rapidly and died about 3:00 this morning.

Decades ago when I was a medical student and then a resident in internal medicine, ward rounds were always held from beginning to end at the patients' bedside. The participants would approach the bed in a group but then would station themselves in strict order. The person who was presenting the history and findings (usually a student or first-year resident) stood at the head of the bed on the patient's left side, and the person being presented to (an outside attending physician or member of the faculty) was directly opposite; the remaining residents and students disposed themselves in between. Presenting and discussing at the bedside occasioned elaborate euphemisms, designed neither to inform nor to offend the patient: "mitotic disease" for cancer, "ethanol" for liquor, "preordained" for incurable, and many others. There were no hands in pockets, everybody paid undeviating attention, and we rocked back and forth from heels to toes to keep our blood circulating because we were on our feet and often standing in one place for a long time.

Times have changed and with them the style and formality of ward rounds. More time is now spent lolling about in a conference room far from the patients, mulling over x-rays and reviewing laboratory test results. This relocation has been justified out of concern that case presentations at the bedside can make patients uncomfortable. The results of a recent study, however, showed that from the patient's perspective, bedside presentations were at least as good as those in conference rooms and may even be preferable.[1] At least in the ICUs at SFGH we still make rounds on our feet, standing outside the room of each patient, one by one, as the facts are described, and then we all go in to examine the person. During the presentation, I usually position myself so that I can study the patient through the door or large window. Just by watching, you can assess patients' consciousness, tell whether they are frightened or in pain, observe their pattern of breathing, learn if they are coughing, check their heart rate, blood pressure, and electrocardiogram on the bedside monitor, and pick up other valuable tips.

Today as we walk up to the room of our first patient, I get a good look at him through the window. He is wearing a baby-blue crepe paper hat that enshrouds all but a few snarls of unkempt hair. He is also wide awake and aggressively complaining to the nurse that the scrambled eggs she served him for breakfast were cold. These are unmistakable signs that he is a homeless person who has been treated for lice infestation and that he is ready to leave the unit.

The patient I am watching, our only new one during the last twenty-four hours, is Wallace Lightfoot, a forty-three-year-old transient who is known to many of the staff but not to me. He is familiar because he has had numerous visits and admissions to SFGH and other medical facilities for the usual constellation of alcohol-related problems: delirium tremens, gastritis, pancreatitis, withdrawal convulsions, and fractured bones. Mr. Lightfoot was hospitalized again yesterday afternoon for another gastrointestinal hemorrhage, this one complicated by "alcoholic ketosis." This is a metabolic condition that occurs when a heavy alcohol binge is aggravated by severe nausea, vomiting, and inability to eat and drink water. The loss of fluids and failure to replace them, in turn, cause the body to become dangerously acidotic. Mr. Lightfoot also has had tu-

berculosis, but the adequacy of its treatment is questionable because his compliance with the medications was poor.

When we visit Mr. Lightfoot, my through-the-door impression is literally corroborated. His hair has been deloused, and he has scratch marks from lice bites all over his body. Still in the clutches of alcohol, he smells strongly of cheap wine and is a little tremulous, but his physical examination is otherwise unexpectedly normal. He must have a strong constitution to withstand the powerful abuse he puts his body through. The most ominous finding is that his new chest x-ray, in comparison with previous films, shows that the abnormalities from his "old" tuberculosis have clearly worsened. But there is no reason to keep Mr. Lightfoot any longer in the ICU, so we make arrangements to transfer him to a special isolation room in one of our medical wards where studies will be carried out to determine whether his tuberculosis has reactivated.

Wallace Lightfoot stayed only one more day at SFGH, mainly wheedling tranquilizers from the nurses to soothe his worsening withdrawal from alcohol. He refused to have an endoscopy to identify the source of his bleeding, and he continually threatened to leave. After a consultant psychiatrist determined that Mr. Lightfoot was rational and could not be held against his wishes, he was allowed to sign himself out of the hospital against medical advice, even though the workup for tuberculosis was incomplete. Microscopic examination of two samples of his sputum did not show bacteria suggestive of tuberculosis. Three weeks later, however, a culture of one of the same specimens was reported as growing *Mycobacterium tuberculosis*, thus confirming the diagnosis. Cultures are more reliable than microscopic examination for diagnosing tuberculosis when only a few germs are present in the specimen. Fortunately, his tubercle bacilli remain susceptible to the standard antituberculosis medications he had been treated with originally. Had he developed a multiresistant strain of *M. tuberculosis*, as can happen with people whose treatment is irregular, his retreatment regimen would have been much more complicated and costly.

A health worker went out looking for Mr. Lightfoot and enrolled him in a special program in which his transportation to the SFGH Tuberculosis Clinic is paid for. And he receives a free lunch to top off his antituberculosis medications. Should he fail to show up despite these enticements, an assistant who knows his haunts will track him down Monday through Friday, give him his medications, and watch him swallow them. This is the new and effective way of treating tuberculosis called DOT, for Directly Observed Therapy. It cures recalcitrant patients and ensures they will not spread their infections to others.

Next, we visit Amos Younger, who was admitted the night before last for a generous gastrointestinal hemorrhage. Yesterday the gastroenterologists noted that the esophageal varices they had discovered when they endoscoped him five months ago were unchanged and did not appear to be bleeding; in addition, the stomach ulcers they had seen at the same time were now gone. But when the endoscope was passed through the outlet of his stomach into the first portion of the small intestine, the duodenum, the crowd hovering around the television monitor could see two angry ulcers, each about one inch in diameter, eating their way into his intestinal wall. At the bottom of one crater a partially eroded artery was squirting a small jet of bright red blood each time his heartbeat sent a pulse of blood into the vessel. Three injections of adrenaline into the tissue surrounding the artery made it constrict, and the bleeding stopped.

Yesterday, Amos Younger received two more transfusions to replace all the blood he had lost; thereafter, his hematocrit was stable. He was held in the ICU for observation last night because when a bleeding artery can be seen in an ulcer crater there is a fifty-fifty chance of its opening up and hemorrhaging briskly again. When we see him on this morning's rounds there are no signs of further bleeding, so we transfer him to another ward.

Then we go to see Jean-Claude Lebrun, our patient with AIDS and Pneumocystis carinii *pneumonia, who continues to amaze us. Yesterday, he had a trial to see if he could breathe by himself, and he sailed through without the slightest hitch. He was extubated in the early afternoon. On my visit to the unit before I went home last night, I saw him sitting in a chair chattering animatedly, but in a creaky voice, with several of his friends, a well-dressed group of gay men in their mid-thirties. This morning, when I listen to his lungs, they sound more water-logged, and his chest x-ray is also a little worse than before. These are not major setbacks for the moment, but they might be harbingers of trouble. Nevertheless, because he no longer requires intensive care, we decide to send him to our AIDS ward. "Does this mean you've given up on me?" he asks.*

Remembering that when I first saw him I thought he had a good chance of dying and wrote a "do not resuscitate" order, I pause before replying, "Not in the least; we're absolutely delighted with how you've improved. This is a promotion for doing so well."

Jean-Claude Lebrun was transferred to our AIDS ward where he languished with progressive breathlessness and weakness. His remaining life was tormented by enlarging bed sores and intermittent diarrhea. Because of his distressed breathing and worsening chest x-rays, his doctors thought that his pneumocystis pneumonia was relapsing, so they changed its treatment. He continued to deteriorate, and it soon became clear he would never leave the hospital. After discussions among Mr. Lebrun, his mother and sister with whom I had already spoken, his physicians on the AIDS ward, and a Shanti counselor, it was decided he should not come back to the ICU for another try at intubation and assisted ventilation. I was consulted and agreed that it was a wise decision: we had nothing to offer him except more misery. Instead, he was begun on morphine to ease his discomfort; thirteen days after his transfer from our unit, he died peacefully. It is small consolation that he didn't die with a tube in his windpipe.

The resident taking care of Claudia Jonson tells us that when the attending neurologist was examining her yesterday, on one occasion she seemed deliber-

ately to turn her head in his direction. Natalie Reposa, her nurse during the day, reported a similar response at another time. But when I try the same thing, over and over, there is no reaction, and the remainder of her examination is unchanged. It is becoming abundantly clear to me that Ms. Jonson has severe and, so far at least, unchanged neurologic damage, and that her lungs and kidneys are so impaired it is uncertain whether she will ever be free of the need for mechanical ventilation and/or dialysis.

While gathered around Claudia Jonson's bed, we start to discuss whether it is now time to consult with Dr. Richard Broderick, chairman of the Ethics Committee, to decide if a meeting of the full committee is warranted, to consider our responsibility for maintaining her life-support measures. I quickly realize this is a mistake and signal everyone to leave the room.

The euphemisms we once used on ward rounds are gone from the ICU because the majority of our patients are comatose or sedated. Yet sometimes we expect everyone to be insentient, an erroneous assumption that has led to carelessness. Things have been said at the bedside— like "There's little hope" or "She'll never wake up"—that patients hear, remember, and remind us about afterward. I was taking no chances that Ms. Jonson might be attentive. Families show that they appreciate, without being told, the possibility of subliminal awareness in their "unconscious" relatives, by stroking their hands, kissing them, and whispering loving, reassuring words. Most doctors do not understand why people bother to do these things. Although no one visits Ms. Jonson, I have often seen her nurse of the day lean over and say something to her; even I speak to her as if she understands what I am saying, and I always give her a pat on the shoulder when I finish examining her. I don't know if it helps, but it certainly doesn't hurt.

This morning, I do not need much of an update on Howard McVicker, who had new abnormalities in his abdomen when we saw him yesterday morning. I re-

examined him and went to see his x-rays yesterday evening before I went home, and I received a report about him from Ian Trent-Johnson by phone last night. After some discussion we concluded that his abdominal distention is caused by a disorder called "paralytic ileus," which occurs when drugs or faulty reflexes slow or paralyze the normally active rhythmic contractions of the intestinal tract (peristalsis), thereby allowing gas to accumulate.

This morning the respiratory therapist reports that since yesterday morning, while all of our attention was being directed at Mr. McVicker's abdomen, she and her colleagues made considerable progress in diminishing the ventilator assistance of his breathing.

After seeing Howard McVicker, we visit his counterpart, Francis Zohman, whose acne and lungs are about the same. His oxygenation still drops abruptly but improves after removal by vigorous suctioning of the thick greenish sputum that is becoming more blood-tinged. As I requested yesterday, Ian Trent-Johnson has had the nose and throat surgeons consult on Mr. Zohman, and they agreed with our assessment that it is time for him to have a tracheotomy. Not only that, they have scheduled the operation later this morning, after obtaining Mr. Zohman's consent and expecting our approval. We give it readily because there is no reason to delay. After we tell Mr. Zohman, once again, exactly what will happen, he nods eagerly and scribbles a clumsy note using his left hand, because there is a cannula in an artery in his right wrist, that says, "Let's go for it."

Next, we go to see our two patients downstairs. The first is Gertrude Davies, whom we extubated yesterday afternoon. Needless to say, she is overjoyed to have that "damn tube" out of her gullet. Her other (nonrespiratory) muscles are getting stronger too. Yesterday she sat in a chair for a few hours. The physi-

cal therapists have already begun to exercise her limbs, and she is ready for transfer to a medical ward. As part of my farewell, I try to scold her into a sense that she should take better care of herself after she leaves. To my amazement, she has a chastened air, as if she just might.

After she left the ICU, Gertrude Davies spent six more days in the hospital gaining strength and weight. But new x-rays of her shoulder showed no indication that the fractured bones in her upper arm were beginning to unite. Similarly, neither the wound in her shoulder nor the surgical incision in her abdominal wall was healing. Her convalescence would be prolonged, but could be safely carried out elsewhere, with regular visits to the clinic. Her husband never came to visit her and did not respond to calls from Clare Brownstein, the social worker. "He gave up on me long ago," Mrs. Davies finally revealed. Clare arranged for Mrs. Davies to be transferred to a nursing home.

Finally, we walk to a nearby room to see our last patient of the morning, Alexandra Papandreo, who has made substantial progress. She breathed by herself for fourteen hours yesterday, and then was rested overnight with minimum support from the ventilator. At 6:00 this morning, she was again disconnected from the machine. When we see her, she has breathed nicely on her own for four hours. She is much calmer, her lungs are less wheezy than when we listened to them yesterday, and her chest x-ray is unchanged. The two transfusions she received have raised her hematocrit to a reasonable level. All is going well.

Alexandra Papandreo has passed the ultimate test of breathing by herself for a long time and is ready for extubation. I am uneasy, though, because as Howard McVicker and Francis Zohman have proven, patients with unstable asthma can deteriorate suddenly, severely, and without warning. Fully expecting the worst to happen, I nonetheless instruct the respiratory therapist to take out her endotracheal tube.

Yesterday evening when I pulled my car into the garage, I got an unmistakable message from our cat Walter: "You're spending too much time at the hospital." He was waiting in the entry alcove, as usual, and greeted me with "it's-about-time" meows. But after we reached the top of the stairs that lead into the front room, where I always give him a good scratch, I noticed he had collected and laid out, side by side, three of the little balls of yarn that he loves to play with, and that I toss for him when one is handy. Our house is full of these fuzzy cat toys, but they always end up under bureaus, desks, and other inaccessible places. I cannot imagine how he managed to round up three of them. I threw each one for him to chase and bat about, with his impressive feline quickness. His speed and agility are astounding; I covet them for the tennis court, especially for my backhand volley. But he would not retrieve the balls as he sometimes does. Instead, empty-mouthed, he would thrust his body sideways, rubbing it against my leg and grasping my calf with his prehensile tail. After nearly smothering him with affection, we went up to the kitchen together, where he ate his supper and I drank my beer.

DAY	
‾14‾	*Wednesday*

Having a clinical eagle eye may not be as indispensable now as it used to be, though it still helps. There was a time when practically the only way of making a correct diagnosis was by finding a definitive abnormality during the physical examination. The master diagnostician Sir Matthew Hope, in Henry James's *The Wings of the Dove*, must have had this talent. There was no other way at the time. When I was a medical student and resident, I met a few old-timers who could diagnose scurvy (vitamin C deficiency) by spotting a telltale "corkscrew hair," and who could recognize myxedema (low thyroid function) from the patient's coarse-textured skin and sparse eyebrows. Today these diagnoses are made by measuring the levels in the blood of ascorbic acid and thyroid hormone, respectively, permitting a more reliable and earlier diagnosis than the presence of abnormalities on physical examination.

Phenomenal improvements in the technical aspects of medicine have led physicians, especially young residents and clinical fellows, to a reverence for and reliance on the results of laboratory tests and x-rays. This faith is often misplaced at the expense of simple clinical examination.

During ward rounds in the medical ICU, the attending physician examines every patient every day, and regularly turns up abnormalities that have been overlooked or misinterpreted: an enlarged lymph node or spleen, a new or changed heart murmur, characteristic skin lesions, air bubbles in the neck, tenderness in the belly, or a lump somewhere. That is why we keep looking, listening, and feeling; sooner or later, it pays off, as it does this morning, by clarifying Mr. McVicker's confusing x-ray findings.

Ella Andrews, once again challenged to the limits of her good nature, has admitted three new patients during the last twenty-four hours. All are unusually sick, and all are variations on a familiar theme: complications of intravenous drug abuse. As I have mentioned, we see more of these diseases than a private hospital and like to believe we are inured to them. Nonetheless, three patients at once is a dispiriting load. The first one we see is Peter Svandova, a twenty-three-year-old man who was hospitalized six weeks ago for infection of his heart with Staphylococcus aureus, *the same deadly germ we recovered from the bloodstreams of Alfredo Fiorelli and Joseph Schwartz. Echocardiograms had shown large vegetations (broccoli-like aggregates of proliferating bacteria and clotted debris) implanted on his aortic and mitral valves. These two vital gates open and close as the heart beats, to direct the flow of blood into and out of the ventricle, the main muscular chamber of the left side of the heart that pumps blood to the entire body. In addition, his aortic valve was partially destroyed, which allowed blood to leak backward from the aorta, the large artery that carries blood away from the heart, into the cavity of the left ventricle. He was immediately started on an effective synthetic penicillin, and after ten days of treatment in the medical ward he was transferred to our affiliated chronic-care facility. There he was to complete the remainder of a twenty-eight-day course of intravenous therapy. After staying only a few days, he yanked out his intravenous cannula and left, presumably to resume using heroin, despite his having*

*received methadone to prevent the craving for opiates that accompanies with-
drawal.*

*Mr. Svandova was brought back to SFGH last night after being found un-
conscious on his bedroom floor. The manager of the hotel in which he was living
had come looking for him because he had not paid this week's rent. A CT scan
of his head showed a large stroke involving most of the left side of his brain. After he arrived in the ICU, we repeated the ultrasonographic study of his heart;
in comparison with the examination six weeks before, the vegetations on his
two heart valves have grown even larger, the aortic valve is leaking more
copiously, and he now has a leak of the mitral valve. He is running a high fever (104.2° F.), he is deeply comatose, and the entire right side of his body is
paralyzed. Numerous small blackening hemorrhagic lesions in the skin of his
hands and feet are clear signs of disseminated infection. He has an ugly pus-
filled ulcer of the skin on his right arm, where several superficial abscesses
are surrounded by dead and dying tissue. Loud heart murmurs emanate
from the blood flowing backward through the valves that we know are leaking.
This morning's chest x-ray shows that his heart has enlarged considerably compared with its size six weeks ago, and that the mild pulmonary edema present
on the film taken only a few hours before in the emergency ward is now much
worse.*

Six weeks ago Mr. Svandova had an infection of his heart valves, "endocarditis," with *Staphylococcus aureus*, a frequent and serious complication
of intravenous drug use, yet it is usually curable with antibiotics. Now
he is paying the price for having left the hospital long before the full
twenty-eight-day course of treatment was finished. His big stroke was
undoubtedly caused when a major artery in his brain was plugged by a
fragment, an "embolus," from one of the vegetations on his heart valves
that had shed infectious clots into the bloodstream. Emboli are obvious
in his hands and feet, and it is likely that the involved parts of his brain
are as dead and necrotic as the visible lesions of his skin. It is also evident
that the *Staphylococci* have been progressively eroding his aortic and mi-

tral valves, and that neither one can close tightly enough to protect the left ventricle. The backward leak through the aortic valve is particularly severe, and now his heart is starting to fail. It is incomprehensible to me how this young man—or anyone—could wreak such destruction on his own body. Yet it happens over and over again. Stimulation of the "feel-good" nerve circuits in the brain clearly takes precedence over survival in people addicted to drugs.

We have already restarted antibiotics to combat the *Staphylococci*, but the only remedy for the leaky valves is to send him for open-heart surgery to cut out the two faulty valves and replace them with plastic or porcine substitutes, a mammoth and high-risk procedure in someone as sick as he is. No one is enthusiastic about this prospect, but we decide we are obliged to discuss the options with the cardiothoracic surgeons at UCSF's Moffitt-Long Hospital, where we send our patients who need open-heart operations.

According to his hospital record, Mr. Svandova has several brothers and sisters, but none in San Francisco. I ask Jim Shotinger to call them after ward rounds and ask as many as possible to come to the hospital. The prognosis is horrible, and there is lots to discuss. We are going to need their help.

Jesse Williams, a fifty-nine-year-old who has misused drugs for decades, was sent to the ICU just before we started making ward rounds this morning. He was admitted to SFGH three days ago and treated with antibiotics for presumed bacterial pneumonia. His course was complicated by agitation, paranoid delusions, and his frequent refusal to let his doctors and nurses care for him. "Get away from me, sonsabitches," he would say, retreating behind a bed or chair. Then, about 6:00 A.M., his blood pressure suddenly dropped and his oxygenation decreased, which prompted his transfer.

We find that he has a high fever, but his blood pressure has returned to normal. We want to send a new sample of sputum for culture, but Mr. Williams cannot, or will not, cough and produce a specimen. We add two antibiotics to the one he has been receiving since his admission to the medical ward.

The last of our new patients, Clarissa Shafer, is a thirty-four-year-old waitress who has used heroin and cocaine since her teens. For five years, she has been followed for HIV infection in the SFGH AIDS Clinic, where she was seen three weeks ago, apparently in reasonable health. Shortly after that visit, according to her apartment manager, she started to become less active and communicative; after these worsened, he called the ambulance that brought her in.

Many patients at SFGH, like Clarissa Shafer and Peter Svandova, are admitted after being found or referred in by their apartment managers, who may be our only source of medical and social information. At first I was impressed that they would keep track of their tenants like that—it seemed such a responsible attitude. My cynicism was restored when I learned that they were nearly always trying to collect overdue rent.

When brought to SFGH two days ago, Ms. Shafer was unconscious, she had a high temperature, and her pupils were dilated and unreactive, a sign of profound neurologic wreckage. A CT scan showed a weird bulging of her right eye from inflammatory thickening of the tissue behind the eyeball, and scattered regions of destroyed brain, with a particularly large defect in the left side. Her doctors called for an emergency biopsy of what proved to be a collection of dead and dying tissue in the left frontal region of her brain. The neurosurgeons also inserted a catheter into one of the cavities in her brain to monitor the pressure and to remove liquid, "cerebrospinal fluid," if the pressure inside started to rise. Afterward she was transferred to the fourth-floor ICU for postoperative care and to us for medical management.

Between the operation yesterday and my visit this morning, she has remained deeply unconscious despite the occasional withdrawal of cerebrospinal fluid to keep the pressure in her brain in a safe range. She is very skinny; dime-sized scars dot accessible regions of her skin; and obliterated veins inscribe much of her body, hallmarks of extensive drug use.

Many people who use illicit drugs intravenously get away with it for years and years before it finally takes its toll; while doing so, however, they wear out all their superficial veins. Albert Monroe, whom we met on Day 4, is an example. When addicts can no longer infuse drugs intravenously, they start injecting them under their skin, "skin-popping," which leaves the give-away scars Ms. Shafer has.

With the aid of an instrument to look into her eyes, we can see a gruesome black lumpy mass extending from the back of her right eyeball into the chamber that is normally filled with a transparent liquid.

I can see right away that Clarissa Shafer has a deadly, fast-moving disease that is infiltrating her right eye and many parts of her brain. I am sure it is linked to her HIV infection, but it is not reminiscent of anything that we, the neurosurgeons, the neuroradiologists, or the eye specialists have ever seen before. Fortunately, the brain biopsy stands a good chance of revealing the exact cause.

After x-ray rounds, we call the bacteriologists and learn that their examinations of the brain tissue, so far, have not shown any microorganisms; other special studies are under way. Then we go over to the pathology department to review the first of their examinations, the cytology slides or "Pap smears," a good way to look for malignant cells. We are convinced by the experts that there is no evidence of brain cancer, a strong diagnostic possibility. But that is all they can tell us, which deepens the mystery. The specimens for routine pathological inspection won't be available until late today, and the slides with special stains for exotic germs won't be ready until tomorrow. There is nothing more to do but to wait for the results and, in the meantime, to treat her for everything we can think of.

Alexandra Papandreo, the asthmatic whom we extubated yesterday morning after ward rounds, is better. The mysterious fever she had two days ago has not recurred, and her episodes of agitation-linked asthma and high blood pressure are less frequent and severe. Given her stable condition, there is no reason to keep her in the ICU, but we decide to transfer her to the intermediate care unit where she will have the benefits of extra nursing care—just in case.

Practically from the moment I walked into the hospital this morning I began to hear rumors that Claudia Jonson has again made purposeful responses by turning her head in the direction of someone's voice. The first-year resident excitedly reported that he had seen her do this earlier, but he cannot duplicate it when we try together on ward rounds. (Is it me? Am I emanating some sort of inhibitory power?) Ms. Jonson has been dialyzed on a three-times-a-week schedule; her blood tests for uremia have improved so much that kidney failure is no longer a tenable explanation for her severe neurologic impairment. Her kidneys have also recovered some function, and she requires only a little breathing assistance. During rounds, Dr. Broderick, head of the Ethics Committee, comes by and, after hearing about Ms. Jonson's multiple problems, agrees to set up a meeting to review the situation next week.

Finally, we are left with our two patients with asthma and chronic obstructive pulmonary disease. We start with Howard McVicker, about whom we get mixed reports. The good news is that he breathed on his own for four hours yesterday morning, and he was extubated in the early afternoon. The bad news is that he was rechecked by the surgeons in the evening. They thought that his abdominal findings might have worsened, so they ordered a CT examination of his belly, "only to make sure." A slot in the schedule finally opened at 4:00 A.M., just a few hours ago, and the films are to be reviewed while we are making ward rounds. The findings are transmitted by one of the senior consultants, who calls me himself.

"John," says the consultant dolefully, "I've got bad news for you."

"I don't need more bad news right now," I reply. "I have more than I can handle. What is it?"

"Howard McVicker's got free air in his belly. Call the surgeons," was his response. Free air in the abdomen is indeed a singular finding, one that generally indicates rupture of a gas-containing organ, like the stomach or intestine, and heralds inevitable peritonitis (life-threatening infection within the abdominal cavity). Free air usually means that an operation is urgently needed to close the leak, no matter where it is.

But Mr. McVicker is getting better: his temperature has returned to normal, he is breathing comfortably without any wheezing, and, now that the endotracheal tube is out, he can tell me that he has no abdominal pain whatsoever. When I examine him, I find that his belly is less distended, and the gurgling noises of peristalsis are lively. The sounds are usually absent or at best faint after a rupture. In contrast, he has robust rumbles of businesslike activity. Nothing is amiss in Mr. McVicker's abdomen. Fortified with this crucial information, we all descend to the CT reading room to check out the "free air" story.

The consultant is still there reviewing x-rays with one of the radiology residents, and he pushes the button that causes the lighted panel with all the films from Mr. McVicker's study to crank into view. He points out a tiny crescent-shaped black spot (lucency) in one of the films of the series and says, "That's it, fellows, that's air." We can all see that it is definitely air, but whether it is inside or outside the intestinal channel (outside is what counts) is not apparent to any of us amateurs.

Other radiologists, having heard about the consultant's breathtaking finding, drop by and offer their own opinions; the consensus is that it probably is not free air.

But the consultant is immutable, even after I tell him that Mr. McVicker's abdominal abnormalities are improving and are incompatible with a perforation. "It doesn't matter what your examination shows. That's free air, take my word for it."

We do not take his word for it, and we leave convinced there is no problem, and so do the surgeons, who had joined us. Fortunately, we had already extu-

bated Mr. McVicker, because this commotion would certainly have delayed it further.

What happened to Howard McVicker is a good example of a frequent and troublesome by-product of modern medicine's readily available high technology: sophisticated examinations often provide information that no one wants to have or knows what to do with. In Mr. McVicker's case a CT of his abdomen, which was probably not indicated in the first place, revealed a "finding" that I decided not to act on, but that could have sent him to the operating room. In addition, the turmoil of going to the x-ray department for the CT study in the early morning, when he would have been better off sleeping, and the multiple examinations to resolve the debate, have only served to make poor Mr. McVicker much more terrified and confused than he already was.

As instructed yesterday morning by our last patient with asthma and chronic obstructive pulmonary disease, Francis Zohman, we "went for it." His tracheotomy was performed in the afternoon. Afterward, he returned to the ICU from the operating room in better condition than when he left, probably because of the extra cleansing of his airways by the anesthesiologist and surgeon during and after the procedure. He now requires suctioning at approximately two-hour intervals instead of hourly, but his secretions remain thick and bloody. When I first listened to his lungs this morning, I could hear phlegm rattling around in his air passages; after Marjorie Smythe cleaned him out with her suction apparatus, all the gurgles disappeared. His abdomen continues to slowly improve. The nose and throat surgeon who did the tracheotomy comes by to check Mr. Zohman while we are visiting him, and we congratulate each other on having wisely decided to do the operation. We leave orders with the respiratory therapist to resume her efforts to liberate him from the ventilator.

Today is the day that Alfredo Fiorelli is presented at M & M Conference, so I have to rush writing my notes to get to the meeting room at noon sharp. The residents have congregated in a semiorderly line to file by the long head table where there is an assortment of soft drinks and five large boxes of pizza slathered with greasy cheese concealing other adornments. I cut in from my privileged seat on the other side of the table, select a piece of pizza that looks as though it might be less dangerous than the others, and sit down. When the time comes, Mr. Fiorelli's saga is neatly described by his resident, and another resident from the audience, who has been asked to formulate a diagnostic hypothesis, puts staphylococcal infection at the top of his list because Mr. Fiorelli is, after all, yet another "shooter with a fever."

The resident also thinks Mr. Fiorelli has endocarditis, but the prostatic abscesses, which are vividly displayed in a blown-up projection of films from his initial CT scan, come as a surprise. The chief resident in urology attends the conference armed with Polaroid photographs of the ultrasonographic studies he had performed to localize Mr. Fiorelli's abscesses when they were drained in the operating room. In these pictures the abscesses look huge.

The only ambiguous and potentially controversial aspect of the case, so far as I am concerned, is my cancellation of the originally scheduled drainage operation, a decision that the urologists strongly objected to at the time. I thought surely they would bring the issue up again to complain about it. But that intellectual dilemma is scarcely mentioned, and most of the discussion centers on the surgical findings, especially the high-tech photos that everyone oohs and aahs over.

In 1969, the Surgeon General of the United States, W. H. Stewart, told the Congress that it was time "to close the book on infectious diseases." This heady requiem was based on twenty-five years of dazzling successes in the prevention and control of several of the great pestilences of mankind. Smallpox was on the road to extinction, and polio, tetanus, and diphtheria were expected soon to follow. Devastating diseases like pneumonia and meningitis had been beaten by antibiotics; others like measles and whooping cough were prevented by vaccines; and even the mightiest scourge of them all, tuberculosis, was slated for eradication. The experts truly believed that antibiotics and vaccines had solved forever the problem of infectious diseases.

But their euphoria was short lived. Only smallpox followed the rules and was declared wiped out in 1977. With that exception, infectious diseases remain the most important cause of death throughout the world, and several dreaded afflictions scheduled for obliteration—tuberculosis, plague, cholera, yellow fever, and diphtheria—are having a resurgence. Moreover, new diseases, completely unknown in 1969—HIV infection and AIDS, Ebola fever, Hantavirus pulmonary syndrome (a new virus of the measles family that killed several horses and two of their trainers in Australia) and prion-induced "mad cow" disease—have appeared, and some are spreading rapidly. Hantavirus, for example, which was first detected in 1993, has now been recognized in twenty-seven states and several countries. Even more incredible is the wildfire extension of HIV infection: the first dozen cases of AIDS were recognized in the United States and reported in mid-1981; by the end of 1998, only seventeen years later, HIV infection and its inseparable partner, AIDS, were known everywhere in the world and had afflicted more than forty-seven million adults and children, nearly fourteen million of whom were dead. The situation is compounded by the resistance of common microorganisms to previously effective antibiotics. In the United States, antibiotic-resistant bacteria are responsible for more and more ear infections, pneumonia, and meningitis. Multidrug-resistant tuberculosis has been a huge problem in New York and other Eastern cities and is growing rapidly in several countries. The surgeon general should have listened to Louis Pasteur, the great French scientist who established the connection between germs and disease, who said *"C'est les microbes qui auront le dernier mot."* As our experience in the ICU reaffirms, Pasteur was right: "Microbes will have the last word!"

We start today with Cesar Fonseca-Santos, a forty-two-year-old chronic drinker who has been in our ICU since yesterday morning for pneumonia, and whom I had seen yesterday afternoon and evening. A few hours before his arrival at SFGH, he had been awakened from a sound sleep by a sharp pain in the right side of his chest that was greatly amplified each time he took a deep breath or coughed, classical features of pleurisy. He also had chills and felt feverish. When he became delirious, his teenage daughter drove him to the hospital, dropped him off, and quickly left without talking to anyone. A chest x-ray showed pneumonia in the upper half of his right lung.

As the day progressed, Mr. Fonseca-Santos's oxygenation steadily deterio-

rated, despite his breathing as much extra oxygen as we could add through a special mask with big tubes on each side like giant whiskers, and through catheters inserted in each nostril. Finally at 10:00 P.M. he had to be intubated. Just then, his blood pressure began to slump, and our "first-choice" pressor medication had to be pumped in intravenously to shore it up.

When we see Mr. Fonseca-Santos this morning, his round, pudgy face is lax. All he will do when I attempt to rouse him is withdraw from my touch. He requires large doses of the pressor to sustain a minimum blood pressure, and his pneumonia has spread to his entire right lung. We add extra pressure to the ventilation system to puff out his lungs and improve his precarious oxygenation.

Mr. Fonseca-Santos is desperately ill and worsening. I am afraid we may lose him. His young daughter needs to know the gloomy prognosis. When she returns to see him after school, I'll have to inform her, although her strange behavior when she brought him to the hospital makes me wonder if she will show up at all. I hope I won't have to call and tell her, because it's always easier on everyone to break this kind of news face-to-face.

The sequence of events that prompted Cesar Fonseca-Santos's admission to the ICU was absolutely classic for acute bacterial pneumonia, but we do not know its cause. The most likely microorganism is the common pneumococcus, officially called *Streptococcus pneumoniae*, but many other bacteria might be responsible. Until we are sure, we can take no chances because he might die before we have an exact explanation. Jim Shotinger prudently started two antibiotics, each with a broad spectrum of killing power, to annihilate whichever germ it proves to be from among the long list of contenders. Mr. Fonseca-Santos's downhill course, despite the administration of antibiotics from the time he entered the hospital, is alarming but not unexpected. Mortality from pneumococcal or other severe bacterial pneumonias is not reduced during the first twenty-four hours after beginning treatment, even with a highly specific and potent antibiotic. Patients die from the overwhelming toxicity and refractory shock already unleashed by the unrestrained infection. It is disappointing that vigorous care of these complications in an ICU doesn't affect the outcome.[1]

■

Maurice Wolf is a sixty-seven-year-old former mailman who was brought by ambulance from one of our partner institutions. He had been hospitalized at SFGH one month ago for an unusual bacterial cause of pneumonia, Escherichia coli. (E. coli *is a normal inhabitant of the intestinal tract, but not of the mouth, which is the usual source of most germs that cause pneumonia.) Because treatment of pneumonia and other serious* E. coli *infections requires prolonged antibiotic therapy, Mr. Wolf had been sent to our affiliated chronic-care facility for continued treatment. After he completed a full four-week course of antibiotics, his symptoms and chest x-ray abnormalities had promptly relapsed, so he was sent back to us for further diagnosis and management.*

When we see Mr. Wolf on ward rounds, he has been intubated, his temperature is well below normal, he is receiving pressor drugs for his falling blood pressure, and he needs oxygen and mechanical ventilation for respiratory failure. In the sterile phraseology of routine medical description, he "appears older than his stated age." Does he ever! He looks ancient, withered, used up. In addition, he is practically unresponsive, and when we listen to his lungs, they sound wheezy and wet. Both feet are swollen with edema. His chest x-ray shows two large regions of pneumonia, one in the right lung and one in the left, and his white blood cell count is considerably depressed.

Mr. Wolf's immediate relapse after a recent long course of broad-spectrum antibiotics suggests that his infection recurred because it was incompletely treated or was implanted in a location inaccessible to antibiotics, such as an abscess or other hidden collection of pus. He might also be newly infected with an antibiotic-resistant germ. Right now he is dreadfully sick and looks as though he, too, could die soon. Until we know exactly what is causing his pneumonia, there is nothing we can do other than support his breathing and circulation while giving antibiotics that cover a wide spectrum of microorganisms.

Like Cesar Fonseca-Santos, Maurice Wolf has compelling clinical and x-ray evidence of severe bacterial pneumonia. But there is a crucial difference between the two patients. Mr. Fonseca-Santos developed his pneumonia while at home in apparent good health; Mr. Wolf contracted his infection while in a medical institution, after completing a four-week course of broad-coverage antibiotics for *E. coli* pneumonia.

Patients who develop pneumonia in the hospital are apt to be sicker to begin with than those who are stricken elsewhere, but the major distinction between "community-acquired pneumonia" and "hospital-acquired pneumonia" lies in the type of bacteria implicated. Hospital-acquired pneumonias are caused by microorganisms that flourish in hospitals, and thus are likely to be hardy, virulent, and, above all, resistant to commonly used antibiotics.

The last of the new patients we see today is a person I have cared for before, Marshall Tutupoa, who is forty-three years old and immensely obese. He has had many admissions to SFGH, beginning a few days after he stepped off the airplane that brought him to San Francisco from the tropics about two years ago. We have never learned exactly how much he weighs because the ward scales will not register high enough, and we have never been able to get him down to the shipping department to weigh him on the freight scales. We guess 550 to 600 pounds, amassed on a fairly small frame for a man, about five and a half feet tall. The oxygen level in his arterial blood has always been staggeringly low and his carbon dioxide reciprocally high.

His admission to SFGH this time was a copy of most of his previous visits. For two weeks he has had a purulent rheum from both nostrils and then an escalating productive cough with chills but no fever. He came to the emergency department two days ago in hopes of getting his medications, including oxygen, refilled, and some antibiotics. Instead, a zealous resident obtained a specimen of arterial blood and, after being informed of its stupefying abnormalities, admitted him to the hospital.

Once in the medical ward, he was given oxygen, prudently only a small amount, but twice as much as he usually breathed at home, an amount that proved to be too much for his oxygen-sensitive brain. Eighteen hours later, his breathing was deeply suppressed and his carbon dioxide value was incredibly high (nearly four times normal). Consequently, he was markedly acidotic and was transferred to the ICU.

A few hours later he stopped breathing entirely and was immediately intubated. After intubation his arterial blood oxygen and carbon dioxide did not improve as they should have. Jim Shotinger learned why when the radiologist who reviewed Mr. Tutupoa's postintubation chest x-ray, which is taken routinely to check the position of the tube, called to tell him that the tube had been advanced too far and was in the main air passage to the right lung and not in the lower windpipe, where it should be. Due to the malpositioning, only his right lung was being aerated, and his left lung had completely collapsed. This was corrected by withdrawing the tube about two inches. Jim started him on an antibiotic for his presumed respiratory tract infection.

When we see Mr. Tutupoa on ward rounds, he is somnolent but can be fully awakened. He indicates by waving his arms and pointing to his throat that he wants the tube removed. From my side of the bed, I try gently to lower his right arm while saying, "Yes, yes. I know. We're already working on it. As soon as it's safe." It is hard to glean much information from physical examination because of his massive flesh. When we listen to his chest with our stethoscopes, we cannot hear sounds from either his heart or his lungs. Palpation of his abdomen reveals only abundant fat. Our interpretation of his chest x-rays is hampered by his bulky thorax and the upward displacement of his corpulent abdomen, compressing his lungs and making them more opaque than usual. We can tell, though, that after the endotracheal tube was repositioned his left lung had re-expanded.

When I see a massively fat person waddling along, my first reaction is "There goes another one, headed for trouble." It is a well-founded concern. That person belongs among the nearly thirty percent of Americans who are overweight and who constitute a steadily growing and alarming public health problem that is beginning to receive official attention. A little extra weight is probably not harmful, and the "normal" weight tables have been revised upward to take this into account.

I am concerned about serious obesity, which is dangerous because it greatly increases the risks of high blood pressure, heart disease, stroke, diabetes mellitus, several types of cancer, gall stones, and arthritis. Next to smoking, obesity is the second major cause of preventable death. But the problem I fret over is that most fat people, unlike smokers, don't realize what they are doing to themselves. The recent discovery of an "obesity gene" is attracting considerable attention (and a glance at Mr. Tutupoa's brothers, sisters, and other relatives during visiting hours supports the belief in hereditary transmission), but environmental factors, like eating and exercise, are also important.

Without augmenting existing prejudice against fat people, much more should be done to spread the word about the perils of obesity. Help should be available for those who want to undertake the difficult task of slimming down. But prevention is what the American health-care system is least able to cope with. It is much better geared to treating the complications of obesity than to avoiding them.

Marshall Tutupoa, who can barely stand up, much less waddle, has what is technically referred to as morbid obesity, with one of its chief complications, obesity-induced failure to breathe. The disorder is often called the "Pickwickian syndrome," recalling Fat Boy Joe, a character in Dickens's *Pickwick Papers*. Not all morbidly obese persons develop the Pickwickian syndrome, and why some do and others do not is poorly understood. Mr. Tutupoa has all the essentials: marked depression of the amount of oxygen in his blood accompanied by excessive carbon dioxide; the high red blood cell count that gave Fat Boy Joe his ruddy complexion; and episodes of suddenly falling to sleep at inappropriate moments, as Joe often did.

Mr. Tutupoa also displays an occasional feature of chronic respiratory failure, exquisite sensitivity to the therapeutic use of oxygen, something he has demonstrated over and over again when given extra oxygen

to breathe. Every time he goes to the emergency department and someone checks the level of oxygen in his arterial blood, the stupendously
low value inaugurates the administration of oxygen, which causes him to
slow or to stop breathing altogether, with the inevitable result that he is
intubated, connected to a breathing machine, and sent to the medical
ICU. This exceptional sensitivity to oxygen also makes it difficult to extubate him. When I cared for him during his first admission to the ICU,
it took a while to learn that we had to decrease his inhaled oxygen gradually to a negligible inflow, deliberately forcing his blood oxygen to a
low enough value that he would finally start to breathe by himself. Then
we could take the tube out. Knowing all this background information
helps considerably in getting Mr. Tutupoa extubated shortly after we
see him on ward rounds, and in moving him out of the unit later that day
and home the next.

He continued to deteriorate slowly and had several more admissions,
each requiring intubation and treatment in the ICU. He undoubtedly
held the local SFGH record for number of times intubated, but the intervals between these episodes were getting shorter and shorter. Finally,
he decided that he had had enough tubes and that he did not want to be
rehospitalized, even if it meant he would die. If he did die, at least it
would be in peace at home surrounded by his loving family. I partici-
pated in the last of several discussions with him and his family, and we
all sadly agreed that was best. Two days after he made this decision and
was sent home from the hospital, we received a call from the San Francisco Coroner's office notifying us that Mr. Tutupoa had been found
dead in his bed a few hours before. He undoubtedly had stopped breathing again, and this time no one was around to intubate him.

*Bad news about Clarissa Shafer, the HIV-infected woman with a rapidly pro-
gressing destructive disorder of her right eye and brain. Yesterday afternoon
Jim Shotinger and I went over to the pathology department to review the brain*

biopsy specimens as soon as we heard they were available. Ordinarily, I am a fast walker. Because I am tall and have long legs, most people have trouble keeping up with me. Not Jim. Though a good eight inches shorter, he set the pace that I struggled to equal. I was aware that Jim is an ardent jogger and wind surfer, and now I know he is a serious, though uncoordinated, walker as well. I was glad I was six feet behind him and could avoid his flailing arms. There was no reason to hurry: the results were disappointing. We saw inflammation, which was expected, but not even the remotest clue to a cause. The pathologists told us that their slides with special stains would not be out "until tomorrow" (that is, this afternoon). The bacteriologists' reports were also unhelpful. They had finished their microscopic examinations, and all were negative. A host of cultures had been planted, but these could take several days or even weeks to grow.

Meanwhile, Ms. Shafer is doing poorly. She still requires continuous intravenous medications to prop up her blood pressure, there is no letup in her fever, and she remains deeply comatose. Again, we have no choice but to continue to support her while awaiting the final results of the biopsy. Time is against us, however. She has not responded in the slightest to our shotgun therapy, and many of the microorganisms that might be found by the pathologists with their special stains have already been looked for, unsuccessfully, by the bacteriologists with theirs. We have to hope—"pray" is not an ICU word—that something treatable will turn up.

We visit Jesse Williams, who required intubation yesterday afternoon for refractory pneumonia. As before, he barely responds to our efforts to wake him, and his lungs sound frightful. Microscopic inspection of secretions, which we were able to aspirate through the endotracheal tube, showed no microorganisms. In a perverse twist of events, we receive a report that the initial specimen of his sputum is growing ordinary Streptococcus pneumoniae, *the most common cause of community-acquired bacterial pneumonia. The residents are delighted to have made a specific diagnosis, but I am hesitant to join them. I tell them that I don't think Mr. Williams's course is compatible with pneumococcal pneumo-*

nia, for which he has been treated without success since entering the hospital five days ago, unless he has an antibiotic-resistant strain of the germ. I say we have to keep our minds open, but they seem reluctant to do so. Why bother? The culture result is positive.

Ordinarily, once a causative microorganism is identified, we scale back our antibiotic regimen to the single most effective agent. But because of my concerns, I insist that we continue the two antibiotics we added yesterday, when he deteriorated and had to be brought to the ICU, as well as the one he was started on when he was admitted to the medical ward.

After ward rounds yesterday, we discussed Peter Svandova's recurrent staphylococcal endocarditis in great detail with the cardiothoracic surgeons at UCSF's Moffitt-Long Hospital. To my astonishment and dismay, they were willing to accept him for open-heart surgery and replacement of his two infected valves. I did not think he was a candidate: it is doubtful he would survive the operation, and there is the added problem of his huge stroke, which they appear to be ignoring.

In any case, there was an important prerequisite: we had to deal with the superficial abscesses and necrotic areas on his right arm, which were swarming with Staphylococci. *The heart surgeons were rightly fearful that such an ongoing extensive infection would pose a formidable threat of seeding his bloodstream with* Staphylococci *after the operation, and that the germs might become implanted on the newly substituted artificial valves. This would be a disastrous complication because it almost never responds solely to antibiotics and would require a second, even more dangerous, operation.*

To prepare him for eventual valve replacement, last night Mr. Svandova was taken to the operating room at SFGH, where the abscesses were flayed open and the dead and dying skin and muscle of his arm were excised.

When we examine him during ward rounds, everything is about the same as when we saw him yesterday, except for the bulky surgical dressing on his putrescent arm. He is still unconscious and receiving mechanical ventilation.

There are no new embolic lesions of his skin or elsewhere, but the old ones on his hands and feet have become very dark and appear gangrenous. His chest x-ray shows persistent pulmonary edema and enlargement of the heart. The results of his laboratory tests show that his kidneys are beginning to fail. There is nothing more to do for the moment, but it is possible we can do a little less. To find out, I instruct the respiratory therapist to start cutting back on the support provided by the ventilator to see if we can extubate him.

After we spoke to the cardiothoracic surgeons, Peter Svandova had his right arm cleaned up as they requested. I have the uncomfortable feeling that if we pressed them, they would accept him for open-heart surgery now, which I definitely do not endorse because he has had a large stroke from an embolus to his brain with substantial damage. We are not sure whether he will ever regain consciousness or what neurologic deficit will persist if he does. He has shown no signs of waking up since arriving in the hospital thirty-six hours ago. In addition, I am concerned about giving him the strong anticoagulant required during the operation to prevent his blood from clotting inside the mechanical pump that fills in for the heart while the valves are being replaced. Anticoagulants are often prescribed after a new small embolic stroke but are contraindicated after a large one because of the high risk of inducing a lethal hemorrhage in the damaged area of the brain. Fortunately, his heart failure is no worse, so surgery is not urgent. I decide to let a little more time go by to see how things evolve.

Francis Zohman breathed with minimal assistance from the ventilator until yesterday afternoon, when the support was removed altogether. He did well breathing on his own all night and again this morning. His spirits have gladdened remarkably since his tracheotomy. This morning he smiles and is happy to see us when we go to examine him. His acne is improving and his lungs sound better, but his abundant bloody secretions continue. He still requires suctioning about every two hours, day and night.

◼

The resident starts by recounting that Howard McVicker has had one of his usual days: periods of restlessness and agitation that diminish with soothing words and reassurance from the nurse caring for him or his wife, who spends most of the day at his bedside, doggedly reading. As details are added, a terrible thought seizes me. Mr. McVicker is metamorphosing into what I call an "ICU Sisyphus," someone whose medical freight keeps rolling back on him, so he cannot get to the top of the hill and out of the unit. I hadn't caught on during the hectic days of his failed extubations, his ICU psychosis, and the "free air" in his abdomen, but it is clearly happening. In critical care as in mythology, a Sisyphus means trouble, endless trouble.

Mr. McVicker's ICU stay, now twenty-one days, has been extended by one complication after another, no relief is in sight, and all signs point to more misfortune ahead, as with the classical Sisyphus. Such patients create problems for all concerned—themselves and their families, the personnel caring for them, and whoever is paying the bill. During their clinical ups and downs, Sisyphians drain staff time, have numerous expensive tests and diagnostic interventions, and receive countless medications. They become "high-cost" consumers and don't often survive. In one accounting of ICU care, only eight percent of all patients qualified as "high-cost" patients, but they used as many resources as did the remaining ninety-two percent "low-cost" patients; even worse, seventy percent of the "high-cost" patients died in the ICU.[2] Mr. McVicker is violating one of our cardinal ICU mandates: get better and get out.

◼

I should have known that this would happen once we had arranged a meeting with the Ethics Committee. Claudia Jonson's neurologic findings have changed and she is better. Imelda Tuazon, her nurse today, could not wait for regular rounds to show me. She is hovering inside the door when I walk into the unit a little before 8:00 A.M., smiling even more widely than usual. She makes me take a quick look at Ms. Jonson before doing anything else. There is no doubt about it. From the far side of the bed, Imelda says, "Claudia, Claudia." Claudia Jonson turns her head in that direction. When I call, "Ms. Jonson," from my side, she rotates her head toward me. When Imelda speaks to her again from the other side, "Claudia, Claudia," she promptly turns that way. As if anyone needs convincing, Ms. Jonson repeats this several times later in the morning while we are all on ward rounds together.

Furthermore, she was not returned to complete machine-assisted breathing during the night, as has been the pattern, but has breathed with minimal support for twenty-four hours. We decide to see if she can breathe completely by herself.

Although we now know how we must proceed and what the Ethics Committee's advice will be—to continue to treat her—we elect to go ahead with the meeting anyway because many people are planning to attend and because the issues are ones that may arise with other patients.

Something unbelievable happened during lunch. Alexandra Papandreo was rushed down the hall to the nearest ICU from the intermediate care ward to which we had sent her yesterday afternoon. After her transfer, she had done fairly well in the step-down unit, with an occasional episode of agitation and wheezing, but nothing unduly alarming. Today during lunch time, according to the nurse in charge, "in a split second," Mrs. Papandreo stood up, started to cough furiously, began to wheeze loudly, and then turned blue and collapsed.

A "code blue" alarm went out to Ian Trent-Johnson, who fortunately was nearby. He found Mrs. Papandreo struggling with all her might to breathe, but moving almost no air into and out of her lungs. Seconds later, an anesthesiologist arrived and was able to pass an endotracheal tube with ease. But then he

*found it difficult to press air into Mrs. Papandreo's obstinate lungs by squash-
ing the recoiling elastic bag he uses to force breathing.*

*When Alexandra Papandreo arrived in the ICU, an oxygen monitor showed
that her oxygenation was satisfactory, but the anesthesiologist was still having
uncommon trouble squeezing air into her lungs. Suddenly, Mrs. Papandreo's
blood pressure and pulse both disappeared, and she again turned blue. Ian was
unable to hear the usual sounds of air entering either of her lungs. Tiny air
bubbles appeared under the skin of the left side of her neck and chest, indicating
she had probably ruptured her left lung. A tube was hastily introduced into the
cavity on that side, and a loud shwoosh of air gushed out of her chest. But it was
too late. She never regained a pulse or blood pressure and was pronounced dead
after a fruitless attempt at resuscitation.*

*Her family had not yet arrived. I had been called and entered the room just
as the chest tube was being inserted, but all I could do was stand there helplessly
until the end. Then, the residents gathered round me, and we agonized about
what could have happened when she had been doing so well. We discussed it from
every angle: there was no obvious explanation.*

Asthma can surely kill people, but not in thirty minutes and not while
the patient is receiving the best possible medical care in an ICU. We
were anxious for a postmortem examination, but Mrs. Papandreo's frantic husband and children, who rushed in too late, refused at first to give
their permission. The medical student who had cared for her finally persuaded the family, with whom he had great rapport, to allow us to go
ahead. The results were astonishing. Although some of the findings
were expected, the cause of death came as a complete shock.

The autopsy showed that there were collections of air under the skin
of the chest and abdomen and even down in the groin. The air came
from a tear in her left lung, which had burst and collapsed. Both lungs
showed evidence of long-term smoking, black deposits of tar, and destruction from emphysema. When the windpipe was cut open for inspection, the prosector observed fragments of orange vegetable material "consistent with carrot." When the two central airways to the right

and left lungs were examined, the one leading to the left lung was noted to contain a little mucus, but the main air passage to the right lung was occluded by a large chunk of orange-red carrot, which looked to me to be over an inch long. These unexpected observations changed the cause of death from disease to accident, requiring by law that the autopsy at SFGH be terminated. The case was turned over to the San Francisco Coroner.

Alexandra Papandreo choked on a carrot. This triggered her instant asthma attack and led to the events that killed her. Weeks later, when all the information became available, the saga was discussed in detail at M & M. I asked if Mrs. Papandreo might have aspirated the pieces of carrot at home, speculating that this might have been what caused her asthma to worsen and led to her hospitalization. The pathologist said that was not possible because microscopic examination proved that the carrot was newly inhaled and had not been in the air passages for several days. We know the large piece didn't come from the SFGH kitchen because carrots here are served diced, not whole. She had gotten hold of a carrot somehow, perhaps from a well-meaning visitor.

DAY 16	*Friday*

When I walk into the 5R unit this morning, I guess from the huge smile on Ian Trent-Johnson's face that something fabulous has happened. Indeed it has: there have been no new admissions to our ICU service during the last twenty-four hours. None at all. Ian has had a busy night, but in keeping with his studious habits, he managed to spend time in the medical library where he read up on Group A streptococcal infections. He spurns the "orthopedic library," which is where the housestaff go to lift weights and exercise. We still have eight very sick patients, but the lack of new ones will give us ample time to reflect on our holdovers, and, for once, I might be able to do a little deliberate teaching. We set off on rounds with the goal of finishing by 9:30 A.M., so the residents will get to Morning Report, one of their favorite teaching sessions, for the first time this week, and I'll have an hour free to catch up on a few of the many items that have accumulated on my desk since the month began.

Ian went to the library to learn more about Cesar Fonseca-Santos, who has been in deep shock ever since he was intubated the night before last. This morning he can barely be roused from his languor, and his pneumonia has spread from the entire right lung to the lower part of his left lung. Ian announces, "One of the techs in the bacty lab called yesterday afternoon to report that a Group A Streptococcus pyogenes has been isolated from all three of Cesar's blood cultures." This is crucial information. Even though one of the antibiotics that Mr. Fonseca-Santos has been receiving is highly effective against this particular type of Streptococcus, we switch to penicillin, which, as Ian reaffirms, remains the best treatment. We decide to continue the other broad-spectrum antibiotic because of the possibility he has a mixed infection. If he does, and we were to stop this medication, he would surely die.

Group A *Streptococcus pyogenes* is a fiendish microbe that is surfacing with renewed virulence in many parts of the world. The germ was ubiquitous before and just after the Second World War, when most people or their families encountered the organism in one of its many guises. My sister had scarlet fever, which caused our whole family to be quarantined for six weeks, and I had a bad "strep tonsillitis," which led to an abscess in the back of my throat and an unforgettable drainage procedure.

In the 1960s and 1970s, the prevalence of Group A streptococcal infections dramatically decreased, but the decline was short lived before the germ rebounded in new and dangerous forms. In 1990, the "Muppeteer" Jim Hensen succumbed to "flesh-eating disease" (necrotizing fasciitis, a fulminating infection of muscles and their surrounding sheaths), an event that attracted considerable media attention because of the speed with which this formerly healthy person died. Another recent type of streptococcal infection is "toxic shock syndrome" (a precipitous drop in blood pressure, a raging fever, and, within hours, failure of several organs).

Cesar Fonseca-Santos has neither of these new complications of Group A streptococcal infection. He has old-fashioned pneumonia. He does, however, manifest a prominent feature of necrotizing fasciitis and toxic shock: refractory low blood pressure. The longer it lasts, the more ill-fated the outcome. We want to keep Mr. Fonseca-Santos's daughter informed about his worsening condition. I wonder how she will take the news. She goes to school all day and then drops by for a very brief visit. I have no idea how much she cares for him.

Peter Svandova is now in his third day of treatment for recurrent staphylococcal endocarditis. Yesterday afternoon, after a successful four-hour trial to see if he could breathe without the ventilator, he was extubated. Since then, he has breathed by himself but with a strikingly abnormal pattern called "Cheyne-Stokes respiration," a type of cyclic breathing in which the breaths increase successively in rate and depth, then slow down, become shallow, finally stop altogether, and resume only after an excruciating delay. At the peak of his breathing crescendo, as usually happens, Mr. Svandova becomes restless and squirmy, but just with his left arm and leg, because the right side of his body remains paralyzed. The embolic lesions in his hands and feet are now intensely black and sharply delimited from the normal surrounding skin; some of the larger areas are gangrenous and beginning to ulcerate. His family is on the way, and we have to prepare them for the worst.

The attending neurologist has made his consultation before we start our rounds. He wrote that Peter Svandova has suffered a severe stroke from a large embolus to the dominant side of his brain. The likelihood of his regaining speech is poor and of his recovering muscular control of the right side of his body even poorer. This morning his kidneys are failing, and his hands and feet are starting to rot. It is now easy to conclude that Mr. Svandova is definitely not a candidate for open heart surgery and valve replacement. His sister, the first of his large family to arrive, and the cardiologist whom we have consulted, agree that an operation is out of the question. Once this matter is settled, I write an order in his chart that no matter what happens, he is not to be given medications to support his blood pressure if it falls again, he is not to be reintubated, and he is not to be resuscitated. We have given up hope that he can be saved.

Later, more members of Mr. Svandova's family arrive, and Ian Trent-Johnson explains the situation to them. After hearing the full story, they decide that they want all his treatment discontinued, including antibiotics—everything except oxygen and painkillers. They also want him moved out of the ICU, so that they can visit him in a less frenetic atmosphere. Ian calls me at home to convey their requests, and I agree with them. Mr. Svandova is promptly transferred to a single room in one of the medical wards.

The next day, his blood pressure starts to fall, and he dies peacefully a few hours later with all his brothers and sisters beside him. This kind of death delegation is not unusual. Many families, even those who may have formerly abandoned or ostracized a difficult relative, like drug-addicted Peter Svandova, rally around at the end. It can be deeply healing for everyone.

Before I left the hospital yesterday evening, I learned from Ian Trent-Johnson that Jesse Williams, our drug-using patient who is believed by everyone but me to have pneumococcal pneumonia, had done so well on his trial of weaning from the ventilator that Ian had ordered the endotracheal tube taken out. As I have mentioned, there is often an element of mystique in deciding when to extubate certain patients, and some residents, through lack of confidence, leave the tube in longer than necessary. Ian has already mastered the nuances and is appropriately aggressive. This morning Mr. Williams continues to breathe well on his own, and his high temperature has become normal. His chest x-ray is also better. Even though I remain in doubt about the exact cause of Mr. Williams's trip to the ICU, I can't complain about how it has turned out, and I give the order to transfer him back to the medical ward he came from.

We move on to see Clarissa Shafer, the AIDS patient with the undiagnosed disease of her brain and eye, who has continued to deteriorate. She needs more in-

travenous medications than before to control her blood pressure, and her neuro-logic examination shows even worse abnormalities. We now have anatomic doc-umentation of the ongoing savaging of her brain: a new CT scan of her head, taken last night, reveals astonishing progression, in only four days, of the rui-nous process that now involves almost her entire brain. We decide to check once more with the bacteriologists and pathologists to make certain we have not over-looked anything treatable. If nothing turns up, we'll take the catheter out of her brain, stop the blood-pressure-sustaining medications, disconnect her from the ventilator, and let her die. All but one of our extended team recognize that even if we discover something treatable, it is too late to do anything about it now; our dissenter, the medical student caring for her, wants another brain biopsy.

The bacteriologists and pathologists had nothing to offer. Later that day, I met with the chief of neurosurgery, who had assisted at Clarissa Shafer's brain biopsy and who had been following her. We discussed her condition with the attending neurologist, who also knew her well. All of us agreed that there was zero chance for survival and that we should withdraw support. Unfortunately, there was no one to communicate with because, despite a thorough search during her hospitalization, no family had been found and no friends had come to visit her. I wrote the usual "do not resuscitate order" before leaving the hospital that night.

Ms. Shafer died shortly after midnight, demonstrating yet again that once the premise of inevitable and imminent demise has been ac-cepted and the order given to withhold treatment, death becomes a self-fulfilling prophecy.

Once dead, a person's body in San Francisco belongs to the next of kin, and permission for an autopsy must come from that relative. When there are no relatives, the body is under the jurisdiction of the Public Administrator's Office, a branch of the City and County of San Fran-cisco that makes further efforts to locate the next of kin. If these at-tempts fail, the Office of the State Curator of Northern California, which is located at UCSF, decides if the body should be used for scientific purposes. In special instances, such as a genuine need to solve a medical puzzle, the curator will allow a postmortem examination to be conducted instead of consigning the cadaver to teaching or research. Twelve days after her death, the pathologists at SFGH got the go-ahead to perform a postmortem examination on Ms. Shafer's body. The results were startling.

Her brain was riddled with abscesses, and she had meningitis of the delicate membranes overlying the brain. Abscesses were also in her lungs, kidneys, adrenal glands, and pancreas. Microscopic examination of tissue from all these sites revealed numerous amoebas, single-celled antediluvian animals (protozoa) whose natural habitat is water. Our pathologists sent specimens to the United States Center for Disease Control and Prevention (the CDC), where highly specific immunologic staining techniques established that the parasite was a newly described free-living amoeba, *Balmuthia mandrillaris*, which Ms. Shafer undoubtedly injected into her own body using a contaminated needle and syringe. Before Ms. Shafer, there had been only eighteen reported cases of *Balmuthia mandrillaris* infection of the brain. She is the nineteenth. Most of the victims, like Clarissa Shafer, have suffered from diseases known to suppress the immune system, including one other case with AIDS. There is no known effective therapy.

We have one more very sick patient, Maurice Wolf, the recent transfer from a chronic-care facility with a bizarre pneumonia. I still can't believe he is "only" sixty-seven years old; he looks ninety—at least. In an additional, calamitous development, the glucose in his bloodstream keeps dropping to dangerously low values. This feature of severe shock, especially of shock resulting from infection, is occurring despite efforts to prevent it by giving him large amounts of glucose intravenously. The huge volume of fluid has caused his skin everywhere to look puffy and feel soggy, and his feet and ankles have swollen even further. The only iota of good news comes from a technician in the bacteriology laboratory. She reports that a germ is growing from the sputum sample she received yesterday. She can tell us only that the organism is "gram-negative" (that is, it stains red rather than blue, a rough but useful feature in deciding what treatment to use). She promises a definitive identification by tomorrow at the latest.

We quickly move on to see Claudia Jonson, who made slight but definite neurologic improvement yesterday. Her first-year resident proudly informs us of one other notable achievement: she has breathed perfectly well by herself for the entire twenty-four hours, and for the first day in more than four months received no assistance from the ventilator. To maintain excellent oxygenation, she needs only a small amount of extra oxygen directed into the opening of the tracheotomy tube through a special collar placed around her neck. On examination, she again turns her head to the side and back when stimulated by a voice from one side or the other. But she does not open or close her eyes when asked to do so or follow other simple commands. She has not improved since yesterday, but it is much too early to judge if she has reached a new plateau. We anxiously await further progress.

Our asthmatic patient with underlying chronic obstructive lung disease who had a tracheotomy three days ago, Francis Zohman, continues to do well. Like Claudia Jonson, he has also breathed by himself all day and night, and requires only a small amount of supplemental oxygen through the collar fastened around the surgical opening in his neck. Yesterday he was given some ice chips to suck on, the first sustenance he had taken through his mouth for more than a week, which delighted him. Patients cannot drink or eat while they have an endotracheal tube in place, but they can after a tracheotomy because that tube bypasses the throat and doesn't interfere with swallowing. Talking is impossible with both tubes. Most things seem to be moving in the proper direction, and even his acne is better. But there is one ominous finding: his white blood cell count, which had been normal or only slightly elevated, has shot up to an alarming value. We launch the usual routine of obtaining specimens (blood, urine, sputum) for bacterial culture.

To our great pleasure, we learn that Howard McVicker's course during the last twenty-four hours makes it three patients in a row who yesterday had their best days in the ICU in a long time. When we see Mr. McVicker this morning, he is sitting in a chair, smiling, and trying to converse. It is difficult to understand him because his postextubation voice is so raspy and often unintelligible, and some of his phrases make no sense. His wife tells us he is breathing comfortably and hopes to go home soon.

Mr. McVicker looks better than I have seen him all month, though he is still restless and now and then delirious. Perhaps I overreacted yesterday in labeling him a Sisyphus. We'll see. Because he occasionally panics for no apparent reason and begins to wheeze badly, and because he needs a lot of attention by the nurses, I decide to keep him another day in hopes of his improving further before we transfer him out of the unit. All the nurses, who know him well and who have seen him stricken without warning, agree wholeheartedly with this decision.

We finish rounds at 9:35 A.M. Jim Shotinger, in fine fettle this morning, having gotten up early and lumbered a few miles, and Ian Trent-Johnson, eager to describe the saga of Mr. Fonseca-Santos and to relay the fruits of his studies on Group A streptococcal infection to the other residents, race off to Morning Report, which usually starts a few minutes late. Ella Andrews, who is on call and excitedly awaiting some action, stays in the unit to check with the bacteriologists and pathologists about

Clarissa Shafer. I also feel enlivened, having talked to my wife in Paris before I left home, but I do not indulge in the free hour as planned. Instead, I call the attending neurologist to get, firsthand, his impression of Mr. Svandova's prognosis. Then I find the cardiologist who has been following him and we review the situation together. Finally, I return to the ICU and talk to Mr. Svandova's sister until 10:30 A.M., when it is time to meet the residents in the x-ray department.

Last night the telephone next to my bed started to ring, triggering an old reflex, one acquired long ago when I was a first-year resident and used to get called several times a night. Such intrusions are much less frequent now, but each one still unleashes the same surge of adrenaline in my bloodstream. By the time I have finished saying hello, I am wide awake and ready to respond to anything, even when it is a wrong number. My wife scarcely notices the calls; our cat Walter, however, who sleeps on the foot of our bed, reacts as I do—perhaps more strongly. The bell must hurt his ears because he instantly springs from the covers and is out of the room before the second ring.

I awakened and answered quickly. It was Ella Andrews, who needed my permission, as required by hospital policy, to write a "do not resuscitate" order for Scott Stanley, a twenty-eight-year-old man with advanced AIDS, who had come to SFGH about 8:00 P.M. Ella told me that Scott was in profound shock from a murderous infection in his bloodstream that had already been diagnosed. During a routine microscopic check of the appearance of the patient's circulating blood cells, an alert technician had observed a marked reduction in the number of white cells, but she also noticed abnormal specks inside those few cells that were visible. Further testing had proved these to be bacteria—pneumo-cocci. We were too late with antibiotics, though, and the patient had not responded to aggressive measures to support his blood pressure. He would soon be dead.

His companion had insisted over and over that Scott did not want to be treated with a breathing machine or have his heart pounded on, but in the absence of any sort of documentation or written declaration, his residents were preparing to call an anesthesiologist to intubate him. Ella solved the problem by calling Scott's physician from the AIDS Clinic, who confirmed that they had indeed discussed the matter together and that Scott definitely had not wanted to be resuscitated. Although the physician had failed to record this conversation in the medical chart, the information was good enough for me, and I concurred that nothing further be done. Scott Stanley died about half an hour later. Intubation would not have changed the fatal outcome, only delayed it, adding im-measurably to everyone's distress.

Only one new patient last night, and he died quickly. Our census is shrinking. Of the remaining five patients this morning, Cesar Fonseca-Santos, the man with Group A streptococcal pneumonia, is by far the sickest. It is hard to be-lieve that he could become much worse than when we saw him yesterday; he has managed to do so, however, despite the scrupulous ministrations of the two capable nurses who have been with him continuously, one during the day and the other during the night. The pneumonia has extended further in his left lung, and a second, even more powerful pressor medication has had to be added to sustain a minimal blood pressure. Only his liver and kidneys are hold-ing their own.

This is not the first time I have seen a patient with a pinpointed cause of infection fail to respond to a precisely targeted antibiotic treatment for that microorganism. Unfortunately it happens all the time, and one never knows whether the person's inability to improve is attributable to an unusually virulent germ or to a weakened host. In Mr. Fonseca-Santos's worrisome situation, it is probably a little of both. Whatever the explanation, his prognosis is dismal, and I ask again about his daughter. She had not come in before I left last night, but Ella was summoned when she arrived later and managed to talk with her. She broke down and nearly collapsed when told that her father was much worse and might not survive. After she regained her poise, she said she must update her father's two brothers, who are close to him and deeply concerned. In this way I learn that her brief visits are not because she is ambivalent about her father but because she loves him so much. She, like other caring people, simply cannot bear to witness the degradations wreaked by sickness on a loved one.

Imelda Tuazon, who is nursing Cesar Fonseca-Santos today, tells us that his daughter has already called this morning and mentioned that her two uncles will be here after lunch. I say I will speak to them. Imelda adds that one of the brothers is a lawyer. I repeat that I will speak to them, and ask her please to page me when they arrive.

Physiologically aged Maurice Wolf requires an intravenous pressor to keep his blood pressure in a life-preserving range. His oxygenation remains poor, and he depends on the ventilator to boost his own feeble efforts to breathe, but at least his blood sugar has stopped falling. The gram-negative bacteria growing in Mr. Wolf's sputum have been identified as Escherichia coli, *identical to the germ that had been isolated when his pneumonia was first discovered more than a month ago. At least we know that his desperate condition is not owing to poorly chosen antibiotics.*

Then I have a little set-to with his first- and second-year residents when I tell them, "Give Mr. Wolf two units of concentrated red blood cells."

"*But look at him,*" *one argues.* "*He's got edema everywhere. Blood will add more volume and make it worse, much worse.*"

They are not reassured when I say, "*His hematocrit's falling and he's in shock. All the IV fluids we're giving him are leaking into his tissues. What he needs is something that will stay in his bloodstream and elevate his blood pressure. Red blood cells are the ideal remedy, and they will also raise his hemoglobin and allow him to circulate more oxygen, which he badly needs.*"

Then I have the same discussion with the other resident, even though he has just heard my rationale. When the first one starts over again, I call a halt and say sternly, "*Give him two units of blood.*" I turn to Jim Shotinger, who is on call today, and tell him, "*Make sure they do.*" I know I'm right about this, but we have to wait and see.

Next, we see Francis Zohman and hear that during the routine check by the nurse at 6:00 A.M. his temperature was elevated and that it was even higher immediately before we started ward rounds. Moreover, his white blood cell count this morning has more than doubled above yesterday's already abnormally high value. Mr. Zohman has almost certainly developed a hospital-acquired infection, but where? Hoping to find out, I examine him even more carefully than usual but without reward. His acne is better, his chest x-ray is unchanged. One possibility is bronchitis or pneumonia in the collapsed part of his lung.

I tell the resident to send another set of specimens for microscopic examination and culture. We start him on an antibiotic to combat the germs that were recently cultured from his lungs, and we give him two other antibiotics that are active against the prevailing microorganisms at SFGH. These should cover the possibility that he has some other cause of hospital-acquired infection. Mr. Zohman senses that something untoward is happening and looks at me inquiringly. I tell him, "*Your temperature is up this morning and it's not clear why. We've already begun to search for the germs, and we've ordered some big-gun antibiotics that should quiet things down." He accepts my reassurances, but secretly we are all worried.*

We then visit Howard McVicker, who has the same underlying diseases as Francis Zohman, but with different clinical wrinkles. Mr. McVicker's biggest problem, now that he has been extubated, is confusion. He knows his name and where he is, but he thinks it is 1959, and he insists that Dwight Eisenhower is president. After agreeing that Ike was a terrific president, Pauline Victoria, who was born after Eisenhower died, patiently brings Mr. McVicker up to the present and Bill Clinton, and he seems positively delighted to have arrived in the 1990s. But then his mind slips back to 1959, and Pauline, flaunting her singular wide-eyed gaze, has to start all over again. She is wearing a décolleté scrub suit this morning because her usual pristine uniform got spattered with blood. I stare at her neck, looking for the explanatory bulge of an enlarged thyroid gland. She blushes and turns away, assuming, I suppose, that I am studying her ample bosom.

Mr. McVicker continues to be restless, constantly wiggling and pitching around in his bed. His arms and legs have had to be restrained because every time he gets enough leverage, he tries to pull out his intravascular cannulas and bladder catheter. Mr. McVicker's nurses are always relieved when his wife comes to visit because she is good at calming him down and orienting him. It is obvious that Mr. McVicker is a nursing handful, so I opt to keep him in the ICU another day. No one disagrees.

Restraints are essential in the ICU to keep patients who are agitated or combative from harming themselves by falling out of bed or by pulling out their tubes and cannulas. Restraints look worse than they are. But once in a while restraints compound patients' restlessness and make them thrash around even more wildly. We are committed to keeping patients from hurting themselves, though it can easily turn into a no-win situation. Because of recurrent problems with restraints in acute-care hospitals, the Joint Commission on Hospital Accreditation (JCAH) has mandated that each hospital have a policy concerning restraints. To comply with this requirement and California law, we now use a special order form that indicates why restraints are needed and what interventions were tried in an effort to avoid their use; this form needs to be renewed every day and when activated automatically initiates hourly observations by nurses to ensure that the restraints are not restricting circulation to the hands or feet or otherwise hurting the patient.

Last we go to see Claudia Jonson, who has had an uneventful day. Yesterday afternoon, the attending neurologist saw her again and noted further slight improvement in her near-vegetative state. He added, however, that the likelihood of significant neurologic recovery was low. For the moment we have no option other than to continue supportive care.

A little before 3:00 P.M., not having been paged, I go back to the ICU. I want, before I leave to play tennis, to meet Mr. Fonseca-Santos's two brothers and tell them how desperately sick he is. I have learned that it often helps to have the attending physician break news of this sort. The residents do a good job of it, but there is no doubt that families are reassured by a lugubrious face and gray hair. But the brothers are not there, and neither is his daughter. Jim Shotinger will have to be the messenger.

Each year at least 30,000 Americans commit suicide. Elderly men have the highest rate of suicide, but nowadays the largest number of victims are young adults. Suicide is the third most common cause of death among adolescents. But these figures pertain to acute deaths from suicide, not to what is called "chronic habitual suicide."[1] We deal with chronic habitual suicide almost every day, from drugs, alcohol, or high-risk sexual activity.

Suicide raises conflicting issues about the sanctity of life and the concept of autonomy. The prevailing view until recently was that a person attempting suicide did not know what he or she was doing, was engaging in irrational self-destruction, and had to be saved from himself or herself. Suicide was a crime against several religions and, in many places, against the state. These beliefs clash with current arguments in favor of medical self-determination. After all, what greater expression of patient autonomy is there than the right to take one's own life? This philosophy is being preached by the Hemlock Society, and abetted by the notorious Dr. Jack Kevorkian.[2] There is also the widely read how-to book on suicide, *Final Exit*, by the Hemlock Society's founder, Derek Humphry.[3] Physician-assisted suicide and euthanasia have been voted on in the states of Washington (defeated in 1991), California (defeated in 1992), and Oregon (passed in 1994, and finally implemented in 1997). The United States Supreme Court recently decreed that terminally ill patients do not have a constitutional right to physician-assisted suicide but added that the Court's verdict "permits this debate to continue as it should in a democratic society."

Reliable statistics on suicide are difficult to obtain because of under-reporting. There are certainly many more attempts than successes—at least a tenfold difference, I would guess. The successes go straight to the local coroner's morgue; the attempts go to a nearby ICU. Some attempted suicides, such as swallowing a few tranquilizers, are psychologically important but not medically serious. Others, typified by our new patient, come perilously close to succeeding. At SFGH we are good at rescuing people who try to commit suicide with drugs or chemicals. We rarely lose an attempted suicide who arrives in our unit alive.

As often occurs when an exceptional case is admitted, word gets around the medical corridors fast, even on Sunday. I have already heard we have a patient with chloroquine poisoning, news that gives me a chance to read up on the subject before starting rounds. It turns out that the information I am planning to transmit to the housestaff has been preempted by experts at the Northern California Poison Center; moreover, they have added new details that are not in my two-year-old pharmacology textbook.

The patient is Margarita Rojas, a twenty-four-year-old woman who has been afflicted with systemic lupus erythematosus, or plain "lupus," for more than ten years. Lupus is an "autoimmune" multisystem disorder presumably caused by auto- or self-generated antibodies that seek out and attempt to destroy perfectly normal antigens in a person's tissues. Margarita Rojas's lupus started with the typical red butterfly-shaped rash on both cheeks, but she has been spared the disfiguring arthritis and progressive destruction of the kidneys that often occur.

She has been having difficulties with her husband of four years over his af-
fairs with other women. And twice, eight months ago and again last month, she
tried to commit suicide. Now she is under the care of a psychiatrist.

Last night she tried to kill herself once more by taking all one hundred tablets
in a bottle of chloroquine, a medicine that was prescribed some time ago for her
lupus. Shortly after swallowing the pills, she must have changed her mind be-
cause she called her husband at work and he called 911. When the ambulance
team arrived, she opened the door for them, but then collapsed, and they could
not obtain a blood pressure. She was intubated on the spot, and a pressor medi-
cation was started intravenously. On the way to SFGH, it became necessary to
increase the flow of the pressor until it was "wide open." In the emergency room
her stomach was washed out to remove any remaining pills, and pulverized
charcoal was instilled to cling to any chloroquine that was still unabsorbed, to
prevent it from entering her bloodstream. On the advice of Poison Center spe-
cialists she was given first adrenaline and then the more powerful noradrena-
line to counteract the depressant effects of chloroquine on her heart, which were
causing her meager blood pressure and strikingly abnormal electrocardiogram.

Now she is receiving two pressor drugs, including noradrenaline. Because the
ventilator is pumping more air into her lungs than she needs, her carbon diox-
ide is very low and her body alkalotic; so she makes no effort to breathe on her
own. Her face is puffy from the prednisone she takes, there are remnants of her
old lupus rash, and her fingers are slightly deformed by mild arthritis. Her lab-
oratory test results reveal that her blood potassium is menacingly low, another
important feature of chloroquine overdosage. We decrease the amount of air she
is getting, and we increase the amount of potassium in her intravenous fluids.
There is nothing else to do while she eliminates the chloroquine from her body.
It may take days.

Chloroquine is a product of the extensive research carried out in
the United States during World War II to discover a safe and effective
drug for the treatment and prevention of malaria. Since then, enormous
quantities have been dispensed throughout the world. It is still widely
used against malaria, although its effectiveness has diminished substan-

tially because the malaria parasites in many regions have become resistant to it. The drug is also prescribed to treat mild cases of systemic lupus erythematosus and a kindred disease, rheumatoid arthritis.

There is not much of a comfort zone between just enough and too much chloroquine, and the drug has been used by many people to commit suicide, especially in France, after a book published there recommended it. There is no doubt that it can do the job, and it nearly did for Margarita Rojas, who ingested ten times the lethal dose; but now she looks as though she'll pull through.

The second of our three new patients is Adorna Brown, a fifty-year-old woman with sickle cell anemia. She is well known to the medical service at SFGH, where she has often been treated for complications of her genetic disease. She was readmitted yesterday afternoon for severe chest pain and fever. Like many patients with sickle cell anemia, Mrs. Brown has chronic debilitating pain, for which she takes heavy doses of morphine-like drugs at home. Consequently, her body has become physiologically tolerant to opiates, a situation that always makes it harder to control exacerbations of pain when acute episodes occur.

Once in the hospital Mrs. Brown felt more comfortable after she received increasing doses of morphine by continuous intravenous infusion, and she finally went to sleep. But when the ward nurse looked in on her about midnight, she was difficult to rouse and scarcely breathing. A check of her arterial blood revealed a significant elevation of carbon dioxide and acidosis. This prompted her transfer to the ICU, where she was given a fast-acting antagonist to morphine to counteract its depressant effects on her breathing. At first, it seemed to work brilliantly. Immediately after the injection, her breathing increased and she awakened, but then almost as quickly she lapsed back into her torpor. She was then given more of the antidote, this time as a continuous intravenous infusion for sustained activity. It also had the desired effect on Mrs. Brown's breathing, which perked up considerably and corrected the carbon dioxide excess and acidosis.

When we see her, she is restless, yawning, her nose and eyes are watery, and she is complaining of intense aches in her belly and muscles, almost as bad as her sickle cell crises. None of the residents pick up on what is going on, but I have been through this before. Mrs. Brown is brutally withdrawing from her long-standing opiate tolerance, a condition we are causing by our well-intentioned infusion of the morphine antagonist. I tell the nurse to shut off the intravenous drip, and we give Mrs. Brown some methadone to help control her withdrawal. We also order a short-acting synthetic morphine if she needs additional medication for breakthrough pain.

Sickle cell anemia is a genetically determined molecular curse. A single substitution of one amino acid for another in the chemical backbone of the hemoglobin molecule creates a lifetime of misery and premature death. About ten percent of African Americans have one sickle cell gene, but it takes two genes, one from each parent, to cause full-blown sickle cell anemia. These unlucky persons are programmed to form an abnormal type of hemoglobin that greatly shortens the survival of red blood cells in the circulation. The result is severe anemia. Under certain stimuli, especially decreased oxygenation and acidosis, the red cells alter their shape from normal flat discs to irregular crescents (resembling sickles) and form sticky clumps that plug up tiny blood vessels. The choking off of blood flow leads to temporary starvation or even the death of tissues that depend on the vessels for oxygen and nourishment. Thus the potential complications of sickle cell anemia can involve any organ of the body, and the manifestations are protean. Among the most common and disabling are recurrent attacks with crippling pain. Adorna Brown has more than her share of trouble, but she has lived longer than most people with the disease.

Mrs. Brown demonstrates a sequence I have seen before in our ICU: it starts when too much morphine or other opiate for relief of violent sickle-cell-induced pain suppresses the need to breathe. Too little breathing decreases oxygenation and causes carbon dioxide retention and acidosis that, collectively, stimulate red blood cells to undergo sickling and to obstruct capillaries, an event that—when massive—can be fatal. Mrs. Brown survived because her drug-induced respiratory depression was recognized in time and reversed with a morphine antidote. But that treatment produced sudden and intense withdrawal from the opiates that the cells of her body had learned to depend on. It provides another example of the precarious life these sufferers endure. No cure is in sight, except bone marrow transplantation,[4] itself a frightful procedure with its own troupe of nasty complications that can strike any time during the recipient's life.

The Ethics Committee chairman Dr. Richard Broderick, whom we consulted about Constancia Noe and Claudia Jonson, keeps reminding us not to characterize patients such as Adorna Brown, who are receiving opiates therapeutically for pain control, as "addicts." He is right: there are important legal and social differences between medically induced tolerance and illicitly induced craving. Both, though, lead to physiologic dependence and unpleasant withdrawal if the drugs are stopped or their effects are reversed by a pharmacological antagonist.

Susan Levine is a sixty-two-year-old woman who was admitted last night for progressive wheezing and respiratory failure. She says she has had "asthma" since infancy, but because of her heavy cigarette smoking since adolescence her disease has relentlessly progressed to severe chronic obstructive pulmonary disease. She has not required intubation and has been treated conservatively with an intravenous cortisone-like drug, bronchodilators, and an antibiotic for presumed pneumonia, said to be evident on her chest x-ray. When we go to the x-ray department to see the films on all our patients, however, hers cannot be located. Jim Shotinger swears that the pneumonia was there and looks around frantically for her film.

Missing x-rays are a recurrent plague in every hospital I have ever worked in or visited. Because I spend most of my time at SFGH, I am convinced that we misplace more films here than anywhere else. It happens almost daily. I have complained to the chief of radiology, screamed at file clerks, and thrown fits in the reading room. Nothing has ever worked; now I just shrug—beaten by the system—and do what I can without the film.

We visit Cesar Fonseca-Santos, who has been in the ICU for four days and in shock virtually the entire time from Group A streptococcal pneumonia. He requires two pressor medications, but a little less of each than yesterday, and this morning's chest x-ray shows slight resolution of the pneumonia in the upper region of his right lung. He has taken two tiny steps in the right direction, but he has a long way to go before he is out of danger. Just before we began ward rounds, his output of urine started to fall, always a portentous signal.

When Jim, Ian, and I return from the x-ray department we notice that Cesar Fonseca-Santos's two brothers are in his room talking to Imelda Tuazon. We go over to greet them. Jim, who had met and talked to them last night, introduces everyone. I say, "I'm sorry I missed you yesterday. I had to leave in the afternoon."

"Yes, we heard you were off playing tennis," they reply hostilely, almost in unison. I am tempted to respond that they arrived several hours later than expected, but I let it go.

Then I review Mr. Fonseca-Santos's case from the very beginning. Jim and Ian nod in agreement and amplify my comments when they can. I tell the brothers we know exactly what Mr. Fonseca-Santos has because we have isolated the responsible germ from his bloodstream. I emphasize the fact that he has been treated with powerful antibiotics targeted at the microorganism practically from the moment he entered the emergency department. Nothing could have been done faster or better than it was. Despite the speed and precision of his diagnosis and treatment, he is doing very poorly. His chest x-ray this morning is a shade

improved, but all the other clinical touchstones—blood pressure, oxygenation, mental status, urine production—are ominously bad. I finish
by saying, "There's a good chance he won't survive."

The two brothers just glare. Finally the older one, the lawyer, says,
"We're taxpayers. Don't let him die, doctor, don't let him die. We'll be
watching you."

Not much has changed for Claudia Jonson during the last twenty-four hours.
When we examine her, I have the strong impression the first time I ask her to
close her eyes that she actually does so. Despite my trying many more times,
I cannot get her to follow any commands, so we all leave her room uncon-
vinced that she has improved neurologically. In addition to my parting pat on
the shoulder, I squeeze her hand. No response. The kidney consultants say she
doesn't need another dialysis today.

Claudia Jonson has improved beyond our original expectations. She has
been completely weaned from her dependence on the ventilator, and her
requirement for dialysis has lessened markedly. Despite her being conspicuously deprived of crucial parts of her brain, her neurological state
is slightly but perceptibly better. It is likely to be a long wait to find out
how much further gain, if any, she will make. No one is hopeful. Today
is Sunday, and the meeting of the Ethics Committee isn't scheduled until Tuesday. Although I have tried, I cannot justify keeping her in the
ICU until then because she doesn't need nor is she receiving intensive
care. With an uneasy feeling in my gut, I agree that she can be transferred to intermediate care.

During the last twenty-four hours, Maurice Wolf's nurses have dialed down
the dosage of his pressor medication, though he still needs some. We have also

*decreased the concentration of oxygen in the air he breathes with the assistance
of the ventilator. He received the two units of blood I insisted he get yesterday,
and these stabilized his blood pressure. I couldn't resist pointing this out to the
two residents who argued against transfusing him. His chest x-ray, though,
shows progression of the pneumonia in his right lung. I conclude that the slight
improvements in his blood pressure and oxygenation are canceled by the worsening of his pneumonia.*

*Next we see Howard McVicker and learn that he has had a bad day, particu-
larly because of restlessness and confusion. I think his panic and befuddlement,
which were provoked by the medications we were giving him, are also made
worse by his being in the ICU, with its attendant commotion and excitement. I
want to transfer Mr. McVicker to calmer surroundings, but he could not get the
necessary nursing attention anywhere else. His wife implores me to keep him; I
reply we will, so long as we can help him.*

*Francis Zohman's high temperature and strikingly elevated white blood cell
count yesterday warned us that he was developing a hospital-acquired infection.
Despite our search, we have not determined where the infection is or what germ
is responsible. This morning we receive a report from the laboratory that a bacterium is growing in one of the blood cultures we sent three days ago. It is not a
superbug, though, and could be a contaminant picked up from the skin when the
specimen was drawn. We will know more tomorrow. Meanwhile, despite three
antibiotics, each with a broad spectrum of activity, Mr. Zohman is no better.*

One more therapeutic maneuver would be to replace and relocate the
sites of Mr. Zohman's single intra-arterial and two intravenous catheters, any one of which could be the nidus of bacterial growth. When a
catheter is suspected of being infected, blood is first withdrawn through

it for culture; after the catheter is removed, the tip is cut off and also cultured. Changing cannulas is not as easy as it sounds, because it takes
time and is painful, especially for a patient like Francis Zohman, who
has already had innumerable intravascular lines and is running out of
available blood vessels. There is no alternative. I tell Ian Trent-Johnson,
who is on duty today and will supervise the replacements, to go ahead.

Each ICU room at SFGH has its own television, usually mounted on the
wall opposite the bed for easy viewing. These sets are frequently turned
on, even when the occupant of the room is asleep or stuporous from
drugs or disease. Perhaps this enacts the theory I mentioned earlier of
providing subliminal stimulation to patients whose minds are out of order. Only a few major channels are available, so programming is limited.
In the late morning when I am usually writing notes outside the patients'
rooms, People's Court is often being shown. From where I sit, the television screen looms at me through the large window. I'm sure I have seen
a lot more of Judge Wopner presiding over his court than the patients
for whom the show was intended. These programs are a distracting
intrusion—except in early July, when I usually serve as attending physician. Then the nurses often switch to the tennis matches at Wimbledon
because they know I enjoy watching them.

Before 8:00 A.M. every weekday, all three third-year residents get together in the ICU to plan ward rounds and to assemble one of the house-staff teams. This way, they are ready to start when I arrive, a time-saving feature I much appreciate. Today I showed up late for the first time this month, and everyone glared at me when I walked in. But it was not my fault; it was my cat's. Walter skipped out on me.

Walter and I got up at the regular time this morning, and on my way upstairs to make coffee, I let him out and raised the garage door a few inches so that he could get back in when he wanted to, which is usually in just a few minutes. I didn't notice he had not returned until it was time to leave for the hospital. I called and called, and quickly checked his usual haunts on the cul de sac where we live. No Walter. Then I extended my search to a nearby alley that he sneaks into once in a while. No cat there either, but also no furry corpse on the busy street in between. Walter has pulled this vanishing routine before and always made it home, but I was getting frantic because it was past the time to leave, and I could not close the garage door until he was securely inside. Calling as I walked back to my house, I found him nonchalantly walking home and meowing at me in his scolding tone for having interrupted his sojourn. I told this story to the residents as an excuse for making them wait, but I don't think they appreciated its significance.

■

The first of four new patients is Lois Carrera, a seventy-two-year-old former bank clerk, who has been followed at SFGH for multiple medical problems, including episodic bleeding from her gastrointestinal tract, low thyroid function, and chronic obstructive pulmonary disease, attributable to fifty-five years of heavy cigarette smoking. Three years ago, as now, she required hospitalization and intubation for respiratory failure.

When we see her she looks well fed, even a bit on the plump side, but exhausted and terrified. Her lungs sound juicy, and her chest x-ray shows a new region of pneumonia in addition to the partial collapse of her left lung that existed three years ago.

Lois Carrera's problem seems routine. Her well-established chronic obstructive pulmonary disease is now complicated by respiratory failure because of the recent development of bacterial pneumonia. We have reason to expect that after this episode she will return to the same level of activity she had before, and that she will not be any worse for having had another encounter with the ICU. What would help her most is to stop smoking cigarettes. Smoking causes the function of the lung to deteriorate much faster in patients with chronic obstructive pulmonary disease than it does in nonsmokers. Stopping smoking reverses this. The permanent damage remains, but the rate of progression slows considerably, thus emphasizing the importance of stopping early.

■

Our second new patient is Virginia Powers, a twenty-four-year-old cleaning woman with long-standing severe asthma. She arrived in the emergency room yesterday choking and gasping, unable even to speak. After a brief look at her struggles, the physician in the emergency department sent her straight to the ICU.

When we see Ms. Powers she is receiving the usual remedies for asthma, and an antibiotic has been started, should an infection in her air passages be contributing to her distress. This is somewhat controversial, but we often give an antibiotic to asthmatics who are sick enough to require hospitalization, especially in the ICU, just in case they have an infection. When I learn from the first-year resident that he has ordered one of the latest and most costly third-generation cephalosporins, a chemical derivative of penicillin, I plunge into my oft-repeated spiel, "New is not guaranteed to be better, only more expensive. Many recent antibiotics have clear advantages over old ones, but not in this instance." I suggest a cheaper substitute.

The resident, who obviously does not welcome my criticism, sullenly nods, as if in agreement. But her looks betray her thoughts: "Why can't this archaic fogy get up to date?"

Ms. Powers is still wheezing noisily, but she is no longer fighting to breathe, and her sentences comprise several words: "I'm much better, thank you." Because she has done so well, we transfer her out of the ICU. I tell her she should be home soon.

Ramon Bowsman, a fifty-three-year-old unemployed man, was brought to SFGH by ambulance after having a generalized convulsion just after dinner in his board-and-care home. This poor man was already a medical casualty. Sixteen years ago, he had a subarachnoid hemorrhage, a catastrophic episode of bleeding into the narrow space that surrounds the brain and connecting spinal cord. Additional damage occurred during the neurosurgical procedure performed to eliminate the source of bleeding and prevent a future, possibly lethal, hemorrhage. A few days later he required a second operation to relieve the effects of traumatic swelling of his brain. When the dust settled, he was left with *a moderately severe paralysis of the left side of his body, a tendency to have seizures, and the lack of a key hormone, which is normally secreted by a part of his brain that was damaged, and which governs the kidneys' ability to concentrate urine as it forms.*

When this hormone is absent, a syndrome occurs, "diabetes insipidus," that consists of insatiable thirst, ingestion of gallons of water, and urination of similar amounts of dilute urine. To prevent this syndrome, Mr. Bowsman takes a synthetic replacement hormone that he sprays into his nose once a day. Apparently, he has been using too much of the substitute drug, because his body has responded by retaining a large amount of water that it does not need. This in turn diluted the concentration of sodium and other constituents of his bloodstream to such an extent that it triggered a convulsion in his seizure-prone brain.

This morning he is stuporous, intubated, and breathing very slowly. He has signs of his old neurologic deficit, but nothing new. We leave orders to wean Mr. Bowsman from the ventilator as soon as he wakes up more. Once he is extubated, he can be transferred to the ward for further evaluation and treatment.

We had no trouble extubating Ramon Bowsman, and he was sent out of the ICU the same evening, still groggy but breathing well and with a rising sodium level. The dose of the water-regulating hormone was adjusted, and he was started on a standard medication to help prevent future seizures. After eight days at SFGH, he was sent to a rehabilitation facility under the care of an endocrinologist. Soon he should be able to return to his board-and-care home, which he will continue to need because of chronic neurologic disability.

The last of the new patients is Henry Karsdorf, a thirty-two-year-old drug abuser who was brought to SFGH last night after he injected a mixture of heroin and cocaine. Shortly afterward, he was found unconscious on a down-

town street. During the ten hours between his arrival and the time I see him, he has fully awakened but has a high fever. He tells me his breathing is perfectly normal, and he denies any coughing. When I examine him, however, crackles come from both lungs. This morning's chest x-ray shows pneumonia, almost certainly from the chemical reaction induced by vomitus and acid-rich juices entering his lungs from his stomach while he was unconscious from heroin and cocaine. This "aspiration pneumonia" should clear quickly by itself, but we will transfer him to a medical ward where they will make sure it does.

This month's experience highlights the wide availability of heroin and cocaine on hand in San Francisco, which has the highest per capita rate of heroin-related hospital admissions in California and which is always near the top nationwide. The use of methamphetamine ("speed" or "crank") and other illicit drugs, with alluring names like "angel dust," "ecstasy," and "special K," rises and falls according to fashion. But there is always something dangerous—and easily obtainable—on the streets. Whatever the substance, it acts like a thunderbolt on the "reward pathway" of the central nervous system, the brain's G spot. In susceptible persons, these initial blasts of bliss usher in a craving for more. Soon, all normal ways of attaining pleasure are suppressed, overwhelmed by the heightened enjoyment of the drug-inspired moment, and the biologic inevitability of addiction and tolerance sets in. Then the person is powerless, consumed by the need for more of the drug to achieve its rewards and to avoid the torment of withdrawal.

Susan Levine, admitted yesterday for chronic obstructive pulmonary disease, is doing well. Today her new and admission chest x-rays are both available for review; yesterday's missing film mysteriously turned up. The abnormality, which Jim Shotinger and everyone else who saw it interpreted as pneumonia, is definitely present on the initial film, but it has totally vanished on today's film.

Thus, it was not what they thought but a region of lung that had been tem-porarily plugged with mucus, a common complication of asthma that comes and goes much more quickly than pneumonia.

■

Cesar Fonseca-Santos remains violently ill from Group A streptococcal pneu-monia. His nurses stopped the stronger of the two pressor medications yesterday, but paradoxically, while his weakened circulation was improving, his oxygena-tion was deteriorating dramatically. To complicate things further, his urine flow is only a dribble, his lungs have impressive features of pneumonia, and his belly has become distended. Peristalsis is alarmingly silent. His chest x-ray shows dra-matic worsening: both lungs are totally opacified and look as if they contain no air at all.

To some extent this is our fault. Cesar Fonseca-Santos's need for more oxygen and his worsened chest x-ray were caused by pulmonary edema. In response to injury to the delicate membranes lining the air sacs, lungs become inordinately leaky, a reaction called "acute respiratory dis-tress syndrome" (ARDS). This condition is aggravated by the admin-istration of large volumes of intravenous fluid, which we have been giv-ing Mr. Fonseca-Santos in our unsuccessful efforts to shore up his blood pressure and to increase the flow of urine. The abdominal findings are new, unexplained, and extremely worrisome. We decide to obtain an ultrasonographic study of his belly. If that is uninformative, he'll need a CT examination of his abdomen. But it will be risky, and he'll have to be accompanied to the x-ray department by his nurse, respiratory therapist, and first-year resident to ensure that he is oxygenated satisfactorily and that his blood pressure is maintained, goals we have had trouble attain-ing while he is secure in his bed in the ICU. There are no safe places any-where in a hospital, but we have learned the hard way that one of the worst places for patients to be when their blood pressure drops, their breathing ceases, or their hearts stop beating is interred within the hole of the huge donut-shaped CT scanner, totally isolated from medical assistance. It is impossible to get to them quickly.

I pass on all this dire news to one of his two brothers, who seem to be taking shifts, so that one is with Mr. Fonseca-Santos most of the time. Again, no questions are asked, but the lawyer-brother says in his court-room voice, "Don't pull the plug on him, Doc. Don't you dare." He must sense that I have given up hope.

■

What we wanted most to avoid with Howard McVicker happened ninety minutes before ward rounds began. He had to be reintubated. Since yesterday morning, he had been fairly quiet and stable on the sedative we had prescribed, and there had even been discussion during the night, when things were hectic and there was a need for ICU beds, about sending him to the intermediate care unit. At 6:00 A.M., he abruptly started to wheeze frightfully; and when this worsened and he became acidotic, Ian Trent-Johnson reintubated him. He had no choice.

After the intubation, he was given additional sedation and is sleeping peacefully while we examine him. His arterial blood oxygen and carbon dioxide have returned to their baseline values for him, and the acidosis has corrected. Apart from the presence of the endotracheal tube, which is perfectly located, his chest x-ray has not changed. Transfer from the unit is now impossible, and, given the number of times and duration of his intubations, if we cannot get the tube out in the next few days, we will be compelled to do a tracheotomy, as we were forced to do on Francis Zohman. No doubt about the Sisyphus label now.

When Mrs. McVicker arrives in the ICU and sees the endotracheal tube sticking out of her husband's throat, she groans, "Oh, God, it's happened again," and rushes into his room. Her patience is touching: she must love him a great deal.

■

The mystery about the source and cause of Francis Zohman's hospital-acquired infection is starting to clarify. This morning we learn that four of the five speci-

mens of blood that we submitted for culture are growing the same microorgan-ism, Staphylococcus epidermidis, *a ubiquitous germ that lives in the skin and is a common contaminant of blood cultures.* S. epidermidis *can cause disease, and when it is found repeatedly in the blood, as in Mr. Zohman, it usually means that an intravascular catheter or other foreign object in the bloodstream has become infected. We are glad that we changed his arterial and two venous lines yesterday, and we should know tomorrow which one was the source. He has been on the correct antibiotic for* S. epidermidis *and other hospital-acquired staphylococci for two days, though he is still running a fever. Having definitive information has made everyone happier, especially Mr. Zohman, who is grinning foolishly and giving us the thumbs-up signal with his hand that is not encumbered with an arterial cannula. He is a resilient old man who obviously wants to live and get better. Not all ICU patients feel that way.*

We make a quick visit to Adorna Brown, the patient with sickle cell anemia who, yesterday, was in the throes of a medically induced withdrawal from the morphine and other painkillers to which she had become tolerant. Now she is back on her usual medications and feeling much better. There is nothing more that we can do for Mrs. Brown, so she will leave the ICU soon after ward rounds. I advise the resident taking care of her that she would be much better off at home than in the hospital, and to discharge her right away. On hearing this, a huge smile traverses her face and she bursts into boisterous laughter. "Listen to him, young lady, listen to him," she crows to her intense young doctor.

Next we see Maurice Wolf, whose Escherichia coli *pneumonia has failed to improve. His temperature is elevated, and there has been further extension of*

*the pneumonia in his right lung. All we can do is to check his sputum and blood
for other causes of infection and hope we find something treatable.*

*Finally, we see Margarita Rojas, the young woman who attempted suicide with
chloroquine the night before last. Both pressor drugs have been stopped, and she
appears awake and alert. She can't talk, though, because she remains intubated.
The level of potassium in her blood and her electrocardiogram have returned to
normal. There is nothing more to be done except to determine if she can breathe
without assistance from the ventilator. After learning that the charcoal we instilled in her stomach to bind any unabsorbed chloroquine has not yet appeared
in her stool, I decide we should keep her another day, even if we can extubate
her soon. She might have medication in her intestine that could cause future
problems.*

Margarita Rojas did not spend the entire twenty-four hours in the ICU,
as planned. She was extubated about noon, and in the afternoon, when
she could talk without difficulty, she was interviewed by one of our psychiatrists. He concluded she was no longer a danger to herself. Around
midnight, because we needed the bed and could no longer justify keeping her in the ICU, Ella Andrews moved her to the intermediate care
unit. The following day she was transferred to a private hospital under
the care of her own psychiatrist.

Before transferring patients who have tried to commit suicide, we are
obliged to have them seen by one of SFGH's psychiatrists. Occasionally,
it is hard to tell if an overdose of cocaine, diazepam (Valium), or barbi-
turate was a recreational accident or a botched attempt at ending one's
life. When in doubt, we always ask for a consultation. Depending on the
psychiatrist's assessment of any remaining suicidal risk, we send patients
to an open ward without any precautions, to a special medical ward
where they are under constant observation, or to a locked psychiatry

ward. This kind of sophisticated mental evaluation is complex and re-quires knowledge, training, and experience, as in other aspects of ICU care. There is even a "suicidality scale" for assessing depressed patients, analogous to the scale we use to rate the severity of coma. The stakes are similar, too: an error in judgment can be fatal. Some psychiatrists are better at suicide assessment than others. As in all of medicine, clinical wisdom is essential.

DAY 20	Tuesday

The answer to the question "When is someone dead?" has changed during my professional career. At the beginning, we would pronounce a person dead when he or she had no heartbeat and no spontaneous breathing. Now, with drugs and devices to sustain the heart and circulation, and ventilators and oxygen to substitute for breathing, we look to the brain to determine if someone is dead. Patients with untreatable structural damage to their brains—provided they have no drugs or metabolic abnormalities that might cause coma, and are not hypothermic or in shock—are brain-dead when: there is no response to painful stimulation, no spontaneous breathing, and there are no reflexes from the brain stem, which is the headquarters for primitive but vital physiologic functions. Absence of electrical activity from the brain on an electroencephalogram is an additional requirement in some states. Brain-dead patients have no blood flow to their brains, and their hearts will cease beating within hours or, at most, a few days, even with cardiorespiratory support.

The solid diagnosis of brain death is of practical importance: it allows physicians in the United States to legally stop further treatment. If the family agrees and criteria are met, the rest of the patient's organs, which are still "alive," may be used for transplantation. Until recently, this policy was not accepted in Japan, for example, where patients were not dead until their hearts stopped beating. There, because "brain death" did not legally exist, live-organ transplantation was prohibited, to the great detriment of potential recipients.

In 1968, the first heart transplantation was performed in Japan, but the surgeon who did the operation was investigated for murdering the brain-dead donor; he was not indicted, but the long criminal proceedings effectively froze all further transplants. The Japanese parliament finally gave in to growing public opinion, and the second heart transplantation was performed in 1999, more than thirty years later.

When the brain does not receive enough oxygen, as in deep shock or respiratory failure, brain damage occurs in a preordained pattern, and brain death may or may not result. The most recent phylogenetically evolved "higher centers," chiefly the cerebral cortex, in which reside such essential human attributes as thought, memory, social behavior, and sentient awareness, are the most sensitive to lack of oxygen. In contrast, primordial activities, such as control of the circulation, regulation of breathing, and protective animal reflexes (cough, gagging, withdrawal from pain), are localized in the "lower regions," the brain stem and midbrain, which are more resistant to the lack of oxygen. This gradation of central nervous system dependence on oxygen explains why one or more episodes of profound oxygen deficiency may lead to what is called a "vegetative state," the condition in which the brain stem is sufficiently alive to sustain the patient's circulation and breathing, perhaps with the aid of a ventilator, but in which the cortex is dead, a condition in which "humanness" has permanently vanished. The subject of our Ethics Committee meeting at 11:00 this morning, Ms. Jonson, is a smidgen better than vegetative because she turns her head in response to noises. Yet she has been stripped of cardinal elements of her self: how far should we go to sustain this partial life? I personally would rather be dead, but this is not a valid reason for me to allow her to die.

Rupert Shawn is a forty-five-year-old man who was admitted to the ICU shortly after midnight for emergency dialysis. Among his multiple medical problems is chronic kidney failure, for which he is dialyzed every Monday, Wednesday, and Friday at a nearby outpatient dialysis center. He has been paralyzed from the waist down since he was shot in the back fifteen years ago, and now, instead of living at a board-and-care facility, he chooses to spend his homeless days and nights in the streets in his wheelchair. In addition, he has esophagitis, pancreatitis, and frequent episodes of gastrointestinal hemorrhage, for which he has been hospitalized at SFGH numerous times. Most of his problems stem from his heavy use of heroin and alcohol. Because he was stuporous from one or the other, he missed his scheduled dialysis on Friday of last week and yesterday.

When he arrived in the emergency department last night, he already showed the life-threatening effects of omitting two consecutive dialyses: severe pulmonary edema from all the fluids retained in his body and an alarmingly high level of potassium that was toxic to his heart. When we see Mr. Shawn this morning he has just finished being dialyzed, and his high potassium, pulmonary edema, and many metabolic abnormalities are much improved. Nevertheless, he remains fractious and ill-natured. His body is strikingly bipartite. Below the navel, the level at which the bullet shattered his spinal cord and disconnected all nerve traffic forever, it is anesthetized, immobilized, and shriveled from disuse. His torso, in contrast, looks like that of a Greek statue in the Louvre Museum, which art students spend so much time copying—a Hercules with sharply defined, gigantic muscles, enlarged from fifteen years of propelling his wheelchair down streets and sidewalks, over curbs, across thresholds. I wish that his personality resembled his upper body; unfortunately, it takes after the lower half. No more intensive care is needed, so we ask the social worker to transfer him to his dialysis center for further treatments.

Mr. Shawn left SFGH that afternoon but was readmitted to the ICU about a month later for emergency dialysis, and again two months after that, when I once more took care of him. Although his second admission was prompted by a gastrointestinal hemorrhage that required blood transfusions, he had again failed to keep his last dialysis appointment, and once more he needed emergency early morning dialysis. The kidney specialists were even more exasperated than we were. They threatened never to dialyze him again. At that point, Dr. Richard Broderick and his Ethics Committee stepped in to remind us, "Even though Mr. Shawn's compulsive use of alcohol and heroin is the reason he misses appointments and needs to be hospitalized at SFGH all the time, we are obliged to go on treating his acute medical disorders and help him return to his chosen life on the streets."

The first-year resident could not believe what he heard. "That's ridiculous," he muttered. "The guy clearly wants to die."

"Perhaps," said Dr. Broderick, "but you're not going to let him."

We should not have been as piqued as we were, because much of our time and huge sums of money are spent patching people up so that they can get back to the self-destructive habits that brought them here in the first place. Rupert Shawn, trying to obliterate the misery of a wheelchair-bound, homeless life, was simply a flagrant and frequent example of this behavior, and we had let his disagreeable disposition get under our skin.

Our other new patient is Benjamin Christian, a sixty-four-year-old man with long-standing diabetes mellitus who has had to endure many of its tragic complications, including amputations for gangrene of his left leg and right foot, chronic failure of his kidneys with resulting uremia, and dangerously high blood pressure. Last night, his friend Lance, who visits him daily, found him slumped over in a chair and called 911. After the ambulance crew arrived and discovered that Mr. Christian was a diabetic, they placed a drop of his blood on a strip of chemically coated absorbent paper that changes color according to the amount of glucose in the bloodstream. Because the test showed that Mr. Christian's sugar was perilously low, the paramedics gave him some highly concentrated

glucose intravenously to raise the level in his blood; immediately afterward, he
woke up enough to follow commands, but he was unable to talk.

When we see him in the ICU about twelve hours after he arrived at SFGH,
he is still drowsy and unable to converse sensibly. The chemical indicators of ure-
mia have worsened overnight, and his potassium is starting to climb, although
it is not yet high enough to paralyze his heart muscle. During rounds, we re-
ceive a call from the bacteriology laboratory reporting that both of his blood cul-
tures are already growing the same bacteria, a Streptococcus. *Within min-*
utes of entering the emergency department, he was started on high-powered
antibiotics effective against all likely species of Streptococci. *We cannot im-*
prove on that aspect of his management. What he needs now is dialysis to clear
his mental stupor, remove the excess potassium, and relieve the congestion in
his lungs.

Benjamin Christian's low blood sugar might have been caused by
too much insulin, but this was unlikely because, in striking contrast to
Rupert Shawn, Mr. Christian takes excellent care of himself. He monitors the level of glucose in his blood every day, and he knows exactly how
much insulin to take when his diet or physical activity changes. The
findings of a high fever and of bacteria in his blood cultures indicate that
his low sugar and deteriorating kidney function are caused by blood poisoning, possibly but not definitely from pneumonia.

I knew it could happen when we transferred him, but during the busy two weeks
that followed I had almost forgotten about Truman Caughey. Here he is, though,
back in our ICU. Mr. Caughey is the patient with severe asthma-bronchitis-
emphysema who had been in the unit for nearly five weeks, intubated most of
the time, when we started on the first of the month. We finally managed to ex-
tubate him and send him out of the unit on the sixth day of our rotation. How-
ever, the staff on the ward has been unable to feed him satisfactorily because of
swallowing problems and his inability to tolerate a feeding tube through his

nose. The only solution was to perform an operation, a simple one, in which a plastic tube was placed through a hole in the skin and muscle layers of his abdominal wall and secured inside a loop of intestine. This artificial access makes it easy to feed someone as much as needed. The operation was done yesterday under general anesthesia and, as is customary, an endotracheal tube was inserted so that the anesthesiologist could administer anesthetic gases and support his breathing. Not surprisingly, after the operation the physicians caring for him discovered that Truman Caughey was impossible to extubate. After several frustrating hours of failure in the postoperative recovery room, he was sent back to us to see if we could successfully get the tube out.

The sedation and anesthesia have worn off a bit more since his transfer to the ICU. When we see him on ward rounds, he is wider awake than he was in the recovery room. Instead of gradually withdrawing the support by tapering down the pressure or rate provided by the machine, our usual routine, I decide to try "cold turkey," the quickest and easiest way of finding out if he can breathe on his own. We simply disconnect him from the ventilator but leave the endotracheal tube in place. If he needs further assistance, all we have to do is connect him back again. Fortunately, he breathes perfectly well. After a three-and-a-half-hour trial of breathing by himself, we take the plunge and extubate him. His mother, who is at her usual place at his bedside, reaffirms that if we can take the tube out safely, it should not be put back again. This brings back the same feeling I had before, that perhaps she really does not understand the full implication—that he might die if we did not reintubate him. But maybe even her endurance is wearing thin. People give up, relatives as well as patients.

Cesar Fonseca-Santos remains the sickest of all our patients. He is still in deep shock. On examination he is totally unresponsive, and his abdomen is even more distended and quiet this morning.

Yesterday's ultrasonographic study of his belly was unsatisfactory because dis-
tended loops of bowel prevented the sound waves from penetrating deep into
the cavity. We had decided that the next step would be a CT study of his ab-
domen to help discover what is going on there. While the nurse, first-year resi-
dent, and respiratory therapist were wheeling his bed through the door of the
ICU, his blood pressure and oxygenation plunged violently, so the investigation
was canceled.

One of his brothers is visiting when we approach Cesar Fonseca-Santos's
room, so I ask him to step out of the ICU during our examination. Before inviting him back, I remind all the residents and his nurse today that
they should be friendly and welcoming with the brothers, and they
should encourage discussion and questions. But above all they must tell
the truth; they must not hide, tone down, or exaggerate anything. Nothing upsets relatives more than hearing differing reports from nurses and
doctors. If everyone sticks to the truth, everyone will be telling the same
story. I advise them not to raise the issue, but if it comes up, they should
assure the brothers that there has been no talk of withdrawing support.
I tell them not to be afraid to give them the true gloomy picture, because
Mr. Fonseca-Santos is surely going to die, and we must make his brothers understand and accept that before it takes place. It could save a lot of
future trouble from these suspicious, combative individuals.

I address these remarks to the group in general, but I find myself
staring most of the time at an adolescent-looking person, dressed for
duty in a green scrub suit and with a stethoscope around his neck,
whom I had noticed in Mr. Fonseca-Santos's room talking with one of
the brothers during nearly all of my routine patrols through the unit.
What is this kid doing here? Then I make the connection: a medical
student, Paul Dudley. (As I grow older, medical students steadily look
younger. I've gotten used to that, but this one is just a boy!) Ian Trent-
Johnson, sensing criticism in my gaze, which I hadn't intended, has-
tens to the rescue. "Paul's doing a fantastic job. He spends a lot of time
with the family and has great rapport with them, even though he keeps

giving them bad news. I think he's the only person the brothers really believe."

"That's terrific," I say with reserve. "Let's just be sure we all keep sending the same message."

■

Lois Carrera, the well-fed bank clerk who came in yesterday with chronic obstructive pulmonary disease and pneumonia that required intubation, now has a normal temperature. But—and I can scarcely contain my exasperation when I hear this—she, too, has received too much intravenous fluid and has pulmonary edema this morning. She does not look as though she can breathe sufficiently without the ventilator. Because this is always a tough call, we decide to give her a trial to find out for sure.

■

Shortly after we saw Francis Zohman on ward rounds yesterday morning, his temperature decreased and remained normal thereafter. We learned that the culture of the tip of the arterial cannula, which was sent to the bacteriology laboratory when the line was switched two days ago, grew Staphylococcus epidermidis, *the same microorganism that had shown up first in one of his blood cultures and then in several. Even though the germ is often a contaminant of blood cultures and not the real culprit, multiple identifications are clinically convincing. Finding the same* Staphylococcus *on the catheter tip not only confirmed the cause of his infection but established its source.*

Indwelling arterial lines are less likely than venous lines to become infected, but as Francis Zohman demonstrated, any artificial device can be the source of serious hospital-acquired infection. In this situation, antibiotics alone will not eliminate the germ, and the cannula must be removed. We were pleased to have confirmation that Mr. Zohman's infection was caused by *S. epidermidis* and not by its more virulent kindred,

S. aureus, a common hospital contaminant that is often resistant to synthetic penicillins. If he had a resistant *S. aureus,* the rehabilitation center to which we were planning to send Mr. Zohman on Thursday would not have accepted him for fear of transmitting the germ from our institution to theirs.

After his reintubation yesterday morning, Howard McVicker, our certified Sisyphus, improved quickly. Because his temperature had increased, and it was possible that an infection had precipitated his need for reintubation, he was started on antibiotics. When we see him today, he is awake and breathing with impressive ease. He winks at us with great expressiveness. We decide to see if we can extubate him. I tell his wife, "If we are unsuccessful in getting the tube out, or if it comes out and has to be reinserted, we must go ahead with the tracheotomy."

We are finally starting to make a little headway in our efforts to liberate Maurice Wolf, our patient with Escherichia coli *pneumonia and shock, from the ventilator. He breathed well yesterday with little help, and he was switched to no support at all just before rounds. We have eased up on his sedation, but Mr. Wolf is not following commands as well as I would expect him to. Does he have Alzheimer's disease or some other dementia to go along with the senile appearance of his withered body? Although I am worried about his benumbed mental status, we decide to push ahead with his breathing trial. If he continues to do well, we'll extubate him later this afternoon.*

Today is the day of our meeting with members of the Ethics Committee to discuss Claudia Jonson, who was transferred to a medical ward two days ago. The meeting takes place on schedule, 11:00 A.M., with the chairman of the committee, Dr. Broderick, present, along with another of its members, a highly respected nurse who is expert on the psycho-social aspects of dealing with critically ill patients and their families. Also in attendance are the first-year resident presently responsible for Ms. Jonson, Jim Shotinger, Ella Andrews, Ian Trent-Johnson, the attending neurologist, a medical student from Stanford University who is taking an elective on the neurology service, several nurses and the physical therapist who have cared for her in the ICUs, the social worker who has followed her throughout her stay at SFGH, and two people from the Senior Center in downtown San Francisco where Ms. Jonson used to drop by from time to time. Her long and complicated medical history is presented with élan by her resident, and various aspects are embellished by the nurses, me, and others who know her well.

The neurologist confirms, "She has made definite neurologic improvement during the last few days. But," he adds, "her prognosis for much more recovery is slim, and her chance of returning to a life in which she can sentiently interact with persons or her surroundings is virtually zero."

Next, Ms. Jonson's social worker tells the group, "Since Claudia has no family or surrogate to act on her behalf, I have already filed a petition for a court-appointed guardian."

"When will that happen?" asks Dr. Broderick.

"Unfortunately, not for several more months," is the reply.

After Dr. Broderick reaffirms our understanding that Ms. Jonson has left no advance directives as to how she wished to be cared for under the circumstances she is in, one of the nurses reports, "Claudia told me she wanted everything done."

The inescapable conclusion surfaces several times during the discussion. Dr. Broderick closes the meeting by summarizing what we all knew ahead of time: "As long as Ms. Jonson is showing improvement, she should be treated as vigorously as necessary. Once she stabilizes, depending on the level of brain function, decisions can be made about the reasonability of further aggressive support, including treatment in the ICU and dialysis."

As we leave the meeting, I wonder what Ms. Jonson herself would want. Would she be among the seventy-five percent of the people who, when questioned in a Harvard School of Public Health/*Boston Globe* poll, stated they would want life support withdrawn should they become comatose with no hope of recovery?[1] Singular in so many other ways, perhaps she would be among the remaining twenty-five percent.

Every day so far this month, at least one of our patients has been in the ICU for treatment of a disorder related to too much alcohol: acute intoxication or one of its hazards (injury from falls, hypothermia, pneumonia) or alcohol-induced cirrhosis of the liver or one of its complications (bleeding, spontaneous bacterial peritonitis, coma). Other serious problems from excessive alcohol that haven't turned up yet are delirium tremens, pancreatitis, and poisoning of the heart muscle. Overindulgence also causes accidents on the road, at work, and at home as well as several kinds of cancer, and increases blood pressure and the likelihood of having a stroke. Too much alcohol is a gigantic public health problem.

Against this disastrous medical and social backdrop is the mounting awareness and documentation that just a little alcohol is beneficial. It reduces the risk of developing hardening of the coronary arteries and associated heart attacks, which are the most common cause of death in the United States. It's at least as good at preventing heart attacks as one aspirin a day. Even the conservative American Heart Association supports the belief that consumption of one or two drinks per day is associated with a reduction in risk of coronary heart disease of approximately thirty to fifty percent. It doesn't seem to matter what beverage the alcohol is contained in, although according to some (especially the French) red wine has additional health benefits. I was pleased to learn this about alcohol because I truly enjoy my beer when I get home at night; it's my inner signal that the hard part of the day is over and that I can let down my guard a little. There are real physiological and biochemical reasons why alcohol prevents heart attacks, but I think the relaxing part must help the psyche too. This becomes more important to me when I am attending because the tension grows during the month. There is one more week to go.

Cesar Fonseca-Santos is trying hard to die. We prevent that with intravenous infusions to provide a viable blood pressure, mechanical ventilation to replace his inability to breathe, and pure oxygen to make up for what his diseased lungs are unable to add to his bloodstream. Without any one of these measures, he would have been dead long ago. The Group A Streptococci *he came in with last week must all have been killed by now, but we constantly lose clinical ground to unidentifiable processes. This morning his lungs are about the same, but his abdomen is even more distended and remains deathly quiet. In addition, he has new neurologic abnormalities that suggest something has happened to his brain.*

Yesterday his resident changed all his intravascular cannulas, and we added new antibiotics to cover for hospital-acquired infections. Today we'll try again to obtain an abdominal CT scan, although the surgeons will be loath to take him if he needs an operation. If he makes it safely to the x-ray department, we will add a CT study of his brain. None of this is likely to help, but at least we will know where we stand. We are definitely stumped.

Another option, a more humane one in my judgment, is to admit defeat, call it quits, and let Cesar Fonseca-Santos die. He soon will, anyway. But I am afraid that his brothers are not ready for that. They remain in the "do everything" mode, and the lawyer-brother talks as though he means business. In the old, less litigious days, it was the family physician who would say, "Nothing more can be done," and the family, however sorrowfully, would accept this. Too often now, families reproach themselves after the death of a loved one for having authorized a painful, extended, and expensive period of ICU-induced misery ending in death. Too often, also, they wish the physician had been less eager and aggressive and had told them there was an easier and better way to die. I will tell this to Mr. Fonseca-Santos's brothers, but I suspect that they, like many families, are unalterable, incapable now of assimilating what is being said. Paul Dudley, who has proved to be an excellent medical student even if he does look as though he belongs in high school, confirms that the brothers are praying for a miracle and won't consider letting go.

Truman Caughey had a stormy eighteen hours after we took the endotracheal tube out yesterday morning, but we managed to get him (and his mother, hanging in at his bedside) through several episodes of wheezing and respiratory distress. When we see him this morning on ward rounds, he is back to his baseline precarious status. Our job is done, and we'll move him back to his previous medical ward.

Truman Caughey's asthma remained under fair control, but he never regained the level of mental function he had enjoyed before his hospitalization. Two weeks after leaving the ICU, he was transferred to a chronic-care facility in San Francisco with, as usual, his mother at his side. Later over coffee Ella, Jim, Ian, and I discussed Mr. Caughey: was this disaster or deliverance? Certainly we kept him alive, but we robbed him of a crucial portion of his brain power in doing so. Is he thankful for the trade-off? He can't tell us, so we'll never know.

Next we visit Maurice Wolf, still trying to recover from recurrent Escherichia coli *pneumonia. Yesterday afternoon, after he had breathed by himself for over six hours, the endotracheal tube was removed. His mental status brightened substantially, and he did well for a while. But at 3:00 A.M., he had to be reintubated to control increasing amounts of phlegm that he was unable to cough up. Before the tube was reinserted, he said, "I'm an old man, and I've lived long enough. Leave it in only as long as there's a chance." How old is he, really? Does he have an intimation of death? I want to tell him there is a chance, but now we've both begun to wonder. When we examine him he still has loud noises of abundant secretions rattling around his air passages. His chest x-ray looks as if some sort of hole, probably an abscess, is forming in the region of the pneumonia.*

As we predicted yesterday, Lois Carrera, our heavy-smoking bank clerk with chronic obstructive pulmonary disease and superimposed pneumonia, plus pulmonary edema of our own making, flunked her trial of breathing on her own. Later in the day we started gradually reducing the level of support the ventilator provided; by the time we visit her this morning, she is receiving only minimal assistance. Her pneumonia seems to be getting better, and at last there is less edema. We decide on another breathing trial, this time with higher expectations of success.

Lois Carrera did well and was extubated in the early afternoon. That night she was transferred to one of the wards, where she stayed for three more days before going home. Since then, she has been readmitted to the ICU for a nearly identical episode of pneumonia-induced respiratory failure that required intubation. In between these episodes her blood oxygenation remained low, the usual indication for long-term treatment with oxygen to make her feel better and live longer. Though she needs oxygen, I cannot prescribe it for her to use at home because she continues to smoke, which makes breathing oxygen hazardous. She could choose otherwise, but she prefers the progressive ravages of tobacco to the life-saving benefits of oxygen, another example of someone irrevocably addicted to cigarettes. She seems powerless to make any other choice.

Benjamin Christian, the patient with diabetes mellitus and many of its complications, including chronic kidney failure and blood poisoning, is better this morning. His mental status has improved, although he is intermittently confused and groggy. When I ask him, "How are you, Mr. Christian?" he replies, "Wonderful." When I ask him, "Do you know where you are?" he responds, "Mobile, Alabama." The Streptococcus *detected in his blood cultures yesterday morning proved to be our tough old enemy* S. pneumoniae. *Fortunately it is responding to the antibiotics that were started in the emergency department. He is ready to leave the ICU, but I decide to transfer him to the intermediate unit because he is still fragile.*

Next we see Francis Zohman and learn that he had only a slight fever yesterday morning, and since then his temperature has been normal. His needs for suctioning and supplementary oxygen through the tracheotomy have not changed. We are pleased that his hospital-acquired infection is under control and that no new setbacks have intruded. If he stays this stable another twenty-four hours, we will transfer him to a nearby facility for physical rehabilitation and to learn how to talk with a tracheotomy. When his secretions subside and he no longer needs frequent suctioning, the tracheotomy tube can be removed and the opening into his windpipe will gradually close by itself.

According to our decision on ward rounds yesterday morning, Howard Mc-Vicker was left to continue breathing by himself. He did remarkably well, and by midafternoon it was clear that we would not learn anything more by pro-longing the trial. So for the third time the endotracheal tube was removed. Since then he has maintained satisfactory oxygenation despite intermittent epi-sodes of wheezing. Having already presided over two failed attempts at extu-bation, I am not sanguine about the prospects for this one. Yet there is no alter-native to pushing his antiasthma medications and trying to jockey his sedatives gently and skillfully.

Business was slow enough in the ICU that I decided I could leave early and slip in a tennis match. It was a bad idea. I should have stayed in the hospital and worked. I was overwhelmed by a player I usually stay even with and often beat.

My trouncing came because I was totally preoccupied with our patients in the ICU and unable to concentrate on tennis. Between nearly every point, rather than thinking about what I should do next on the court, my mind would wander to Cesar Fonseca-Santos and then to Maurice Wolf. Why were they doing so poorly? I thought about *Streptococcus pyogenes* and *Escherichia coli*. Why weren't the antibiotics defeating them? I considered Howard McVicker and Francis Zohman. What was making their asthma so unusually refractory? And what in the world happened to Alexandra Papandreo? How did she get hold of that carrot? Once, between my own first and second serves, would-be American twists, I visualized Marshall Tutupoa's immense body, and wondered if there wasn't some way to get him to lose weight? I discovered that it was impossible to hit a crisp overhead smash while the image of Peter Svandova's gangrenous arm was zooming in on my brain instead of the tennis ball. At the end, instead of being pepped up, I was cast down. But my spirits were soon restored by an affectionate welcome home from Walter, who jumped into my lap and preened himself while I downed a healthful consolation beer.

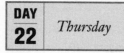

DAY 22 *Thursday*

If people think hard enough, they can probably recall hearing about some now dead member of their family, usually in their grandparents' generation or even older, who had tuberculosis. Then this centuries-old scourge seemed to disappear. Though tuberculosis remained the leading cause of death in the United States as late as the early 1900s, improvements in housing, hygiene, and sanitation in the first half of this century, and effective antibiotics coming in the late 1940s, all contributed to a striking decrease.

But in the 1980s, government funding for the tuberculosis control programs that were responsible for this extraordinary decline also fell, axed by overconfidence and shortsighted policy-making. Public health neglect came at precisely the wrong moment: just as worsening poverty, crowding, homelessness, drug addiction and alcoholism, increased immigration, and the emptying of psychiatric institutions were creating inner-city pools of disadvantaged people, among whom tuberculosis flourished. This urban nightmare was exacerbated by the arrival and spread of HIV infection. In 1986, for the first time in over thirty years, tuberculosis started to increase in the United States. Now it is sometimes caused by a new and deadly supergerm, multidrug-resistant strains of the bacillus *Mycobacterium tuberculosis*. In 1993, tuberculosis began to decline again in the United States, but it continues its menacing upsurge in poor countries, where each year more than ninety-five percent of the world's eight million new cases and three million deaths occur. That's more deaths per year than those caused by AIDS in its first decade. (But HIV/AIDS, continuing its phenomenal worldwide increase, moved ahead of tuberculosis in 1998 on the global hierarchy of causes of death; overlooked in this accounting, though, is the fact that more patients with HIV/AIDS die of tuberculosis worldwide than of any other disease.)

San Francisco has long been near the top of the list of cities in the United States with a high incidence of tuberculosis, largely because of the many immigrants from Asia and Latin America who bring *M. tuberculosis* with them from their native countries. Before emigrating to the United States, people are screened for tuberculosis, chiefly by a chest x-ray examination, but this does not pick up tiny foci of indolent infection that may activate into serious disease after arrival. Also, in many countries it is easy to purchase a normal chest film to show the medical officer when obtaining a visa. Because our city also has its share of addicts, homeless persons, and other likely victims, we nearly always have a few patients with tuberculosis at SFGH, though seldom in the ICU. Wallace Lightfoot had tuberculosis, but he was in the ICU (Day 13) for another reason. So I was startled this morning when a good friend and former research partner, a distinguished cardiologist now taking his turn in the Coronary Care Unit, asked me to see one of his patients who might have tuberculosis of the heart. My interest was piqued by this possible rare complication of a familiar disease. I said I would look at the man right after ward rounds, which should be short because we have no new patients and only four old ones.

First, we go see Cesar Fonseca-Santos, who is resisting all our efforts to keep him alive. His blood pressure has fallen despite the addition of our two most

powerful pressor agents. His oxygenation has worsened, and his body has stead-
ily become more acidotic. Yesterday the CT studies of his abdomen and head were
performed, but they failed to show anything new or conceivably treatable, only
evidence of possible cirrhosis of the liver and shrinkage of the brain. Part of his
right lung is destroyed by an abscess, but we knew that might happen. He is not
going to live much longer, so I ask the brother who is there to call and tell his
brother and niece they should come in soon.

Cesar Fonseca-Santos died that afternoon from the overwhelming blitz-
krieg of the powerful toxins elaborated by Group A *Streptococcus pyogenes.*
His chronic alcoholism did not help his chances for recovery, but even
perfectly healthy persons flout medical mastery and succumb to this virulent infection. According to Father Paneloux, the Jesuit priest in Camus's *The Plague,* it happens because "no earthly power, nay, not even—
mark me well—the vaunted might of human science can avail you to
avert that hand [of death] once it is stretched toward you."[1] There is no
doubt that we dragged out Mr. Fonseca-Santos's death, hoping to avert
it, with all the human science we had. But we failed. In retrospect it is
hard to define precisely when his disease crossed the invisible threshold
from potentially curable, as it was at the beginning, to hopeless, as it was
at the end.

Just after he died, I became deeply saddened even though I had
known it was going to happen. I went in with Paul Dudley, the youthful
medical student, to speak with his two brothers and daughter. I told
them I was very sorry it ended this way, but we had done everything
possible to save Mr. Fonseca-Santos's life. "Nothing was spared, right to
the end."

"We know you did, Doctor," the lawyer replied, "and we're immensely grateful. God bless you both." Then they left, having as-
tounded me with their gracious approval.

"Whew, I'm glad that's over," said Paul after they walked out. "I wonder whether poor old Cesar would have wanted to die like that. It took
forever. Pressors right to the end."

"I wonder too," I replied. "The brothers were certainly clear about what they wanted, but I always had the feeling they weren't speaking for Mr. Fonseca-Santos. They admitted they had never talked about it together."

We agreed it was too bad he didn't leave an advance directive. There are two kinds of advance directives, both with legal force: the more common one is called a durable power of attorney for health care, in which someone is designated to carry out a person's declarations about the kind of care he or she wishes to receive—should a situation arise in which the person is unable to make his or her own decisions. There is also a living will that specifies the extent of medical support desired by a victim of a terminal illness—when potentially fatal complications supervene. "Then we could have been sure we were following his own wishes," Paul suggested.

I am a great believer in advance directives and promote them whenever I can, but I had to add, "Yes and no, Paul. Implementing an advance directive, which usually means withholding or withdrawing life-support when someone is dying and unable to make a decision, is not always easy. Mr. Fonseca-Santos provides a perfect example. At the beginning, he had what should have been a curable illness, and there was absolutely no way of knowing that he was going to die. After a few days, especially in patients with such a fast-moving disease, the prognosis, favorable or hopeless, usually becomes clearer. But it certainly wasn't obvious early on in Mr. Fonseca-Santos's case. Imagine what it's like when the illness is insidious and lingering, with clinical ups and downs, as in chronic heart failure, spreading cancer, progressive dementia, or chronic obstructive pulmonary disease. Then it's even harder to decide when the condition crosses the boundary between reversible and fatal. But you're right. Our job would be considerably easier if everyone had an advance directive. Don't expect to find many in this hospital, though; they have been signed by fewer than fifteen percent of Americans, chiefly by those who are affluent and middle class, though many more would like to have them."

"Do you have one?" Paul asked.

"My wife and I took care of that years ago," I responded, "and our views haven't changed, only been reinforced."

We then visit Maurice Wolf, our ancient postman, who has been in the ICU for eight days and made little progress. He looks so feeble I wonder how he could ever have carried mail. His pneumonia is even worse than when he was admitted, and there is no doubt that the suspicious "hole" we noted yesterday is real. Another has appeared on the other side. We decide to search again for the responsible microorganisms. Also, because his belly is distended and quiet this morning, I tell his resident to order an ultrasonographic study of his abdomen to look for fluid and other abnormalities.

We are relieved to hear that Howard McVicker has had one of his better twenty-four hours. For once, he was neither too deeply nor too lightly sedated. He remains confused and still thinks it is 1959, but his hallucinations and paranoia have gone. His wife, delighted by his improvement, continues to soothe him with gentle words and her reassuring presence. Once she leaves for her night job, Mr. McVicker often becomes restless.

We finish rounds by visiting Francis Zohman to say good-bye to him. He has had an uneventful twenty-four hours, and he already knows he is going by ambulance to the rehabilitation center later this morning. He is thrilled by the knowledge that his transfer is a medical upgrading, proof that he is getting better. Molly Wolford, our head nurse, is there, beaming. Several other nurses who have cared for him during his sixteen days in the unit drop by to offer encour-

*agement and congratulations on his ICU graduation: "Terrific job. You'll be
fine. Great having you."*

*I wish I had a diploma to give him, but I don't. So I shake his hand, now
without an arterial cannula, and wish him good luck. I tell him, "Come back
and visit us; we'd love to see you, but not as a patient."*

*He then writes a valedictory note in jerky handwriting for all the nurses,
therapists, and doctors in the unit who have cared for him—a large number. It
says, "Many thanks for everything."*

*If there ever was an opportune time to see another attending physician's patient
in consultation, this morning is it. Because our regular ward rounds finished so
quickly, I have plenty of time left over to see my colleague's patient, Jesse Jerome, a thirty-seven-year-old unemployed man who uses heroin every day, including a dose just before he went to one of our community clinics two days ago.
For two weeks he had been troubled by shortness of breath, swelling of his
ankles, and intermittent palpitations. When the health worker who first saw
Mr. Jerome discovered that his heart rate was precariously fast and his blood
pressure was low, he was immediately transferred by ambulance to SFGH. After an escalating series of maneuvers and medications in the emergency department failed to slow his racing heart, he was put to sleep with a short-acting anesthetic and intubated. Then two spatula-shaped electrodes were pressed against
his chest, and an electric shock jolted his speeding heart back to normal. A chest
x-ray showed a large heart shadow and fluid in the right chest cavity. When the
anesthetic wore off, he was extubated and sent to the cardiologists in the ICU.*

*As soon as Mr. Jerome arrived there, an ultrasonographic study showed that
the heart enlargement on his chest x-ray was actually an accumulation of fluid
("effusion") in the thin stretchable sac, the "pericardium," that usually fits
snugly around the heart. The pericardial effusion was so large it was squeezing
his heart and mechanically preventing it from filling with blood. This accounted
for his falling blood pressure and presented a life-threatening emergency that*

required urgent treatment: immediate removal of the fluid. Not only is this instantly curative, but studies of the character of the fluid are quite helpful in diagnosing the cause of the effusion.

The trainee in cardiology inserted a long needle attached to a large syringe under Mr. Jerome's rib cage and advanced it upward and inward toward his heart. Soon a spurt of yellowish fluid gushed into the syringe. The cardiologist then aspirated as much fluid as he could from the pericardial sac, more than a pint. After only a few ounces were withdrawn, the nurse monitoring Mr. Jerome's blood pressure exclaimed, "His pressure's climbing!" and it continued to climb all the way back to normal.

Examination of the fluid under the microscope showed numerous single-lobed white blood cells, a finding indicative of an indolent chronic infection, including tuberculosis. Yesterday the fluid in the pleural cavity next to his right lung was also tapped and found to have almost the same number and type of cells as the pericardial fluid. At the same time, the resident performed a skin test to see if he had ever been exposed to the germ that causes tuberculosis. When I see Mr. Jerome today, only twenty-four hours later, a large, firm reddening of the skin is already evident, affirming his exposure to tuberculosis.

It is easy now to answer the cardiologist's two questions: Could Mr. Jerome have tuberculosis of the membranes lining his heart and right lung? And, more important, is the risk high enough that he should be started on antituberculosis medications right now, without waiting two or more weeks for the results of the cultures? My answer to both questions is an unqualified "yes," even though there are other diagnostic possibilities. In addition to treating him for tuberculosis, I suggest a biopsy of his pleural membrane by using a special needle to sample the tissue; this is sometimes a fast way to establish the diagnosis. He should definitely have a serologic test for HIV because he is an intravenous drug user at high risk of being infected with the virus.

Mr. Jerome refused the biopsy. One week after I saw him he signed himself out of the hospital against the advice of his physicians. But he agreed to keep taking his antituberculosis medications, and it was lucky for him he did. Later the cultures of the pericardial and pleural fluids were reported positive for *M. tuberculosis;* his blood serologic test for HIV was positive too. This verified that his tuberculosis is linked to HIV infection.

One third of the world's population of over six billion people is believed to be infected with *M. tuberculosis*. Yet the great majority, ninety percent, of these otherwise healthy persons do not develop active clinical tuberculosis. Their efficient immune systems keep the bacilli in check, though they are still alive within their bodies. Immunologic erosions of any kind, and particularly of HIV infection, increase the likelihood that innocent tuberculous infection, whether newly acquired or ancient, will flare into significant disease. The "cursed duet" of HIV and *M. tuberculosis* accounted for much of the resurgence of tuberculosis in the United States between 1986 and 1992. Also, it explains the explosion of tuberculosis under way in sub-Saharan Africa and guarantees an enormous increase during the next decade as HIV continues to propagate in Southeast Asia and India, places where the majority of adults are already infected with the tuberculosis germs.

DAY	
23	*Friday*

When I started medical school we were told that we would have to master a huge new vocabulary, said to be at least the equivalent of an entire foreign language. During my first year, I prepared and studied flash cards with new, specialized words like "polymorphonuclear leukocyte" and "natriuresis" written on one side and their definitions ("multilobed white blood pus cell" and "excretion of sodium in the urine") on the other side, exactly as I did when I was studying German to qualify for admission. (The foreign language requirement, German or French, was dropped by most medical schools many years ago.) The esoteric language of medicine is important because it enables physicians to communicate with each other about sophisticated, often highly complex matters. As used in ordinary conversation, though, and especially during ward rounds, medical discourse has been radically truncated into a clinical-technical idiom that is becoming unintelligible, particularly to physicians outside the speaker's own specialty and local argot.

Things change fast, and I get caught short from time to time by an unfamiliar abbreviation or new bit of jargon. "SOB" is not what President Harry Truman called the columnist Drew Pearson but almost the

226

opposite: "shortness of breath." I had no trouble inferring that the state-ment, "He was satting gloriously, one hundred percent on two liters of cannulas," indicated that "the patient's oxygen saturation, a routine mea-surement of oxygenation, was one hundred percent, as high as it can get, while he was breathing supplementary oxygen administered at a rate of two liters per minute through a cannula positioned within his nose." But the phrase "She was tachy" threw me for a while, until I figured out it meant "She had a fast heart rate" (or tachycardia). The first time I heard "We lined the guy up," I had to ask the resident what he meant. I learned that it was shorthand for saying, "Several cannulas, 'lines,' have been in-serted into the patient, one into one of his peripheral arteries, a second into a peripheral vein, a third into the pulmonary artery, and a near-line, a catheter, has been placed in the bladder," all for monitoring purposes. I also interpreted the word "guy" wrong, thinking he meant a man. Had he said "gal," I would have understood that the patient was a woman.

The first of our two new patients is David Ignatious, a twenty-six-year-old man with diabetes mellitus, which he controls with daily injections of insu-lin. He occasionally snorts cocaine. Yesterday morning at home he went into the bathroom but failed to come out. After a long wait, his roommate finally checked and found him unconscious on the floor. In the ambulance on his way to the hos-pital, he had a violent but short-lived seizure, and in the emergency department he began a prolonged seizure with furious paroxysms that did not stop until he was heavily medicated with anticonvulsants and deeply sedated with pheno-barbital. His virtual anesthesia necessitated intubation and assisted ventilation. A CT scan of his head showed a marble-sized region void of nerve cells in his "pons," a strategic control center tucked away in the middle of the brain.

Today he is still in a deep coma and has other signs of severe neurologic im-pairment, including the complete absence of breathing when detached from the ventilator. When we review his CT scan, the neuroradiologist has no doubts about the presence of a translucent area within the pons where nerve cells are *conspicuously absent. She is vague about its cause. We learn that a routine* *chemical examination of his urine turned up cocaine.*

During our subsequent discussion, the first-year resident asks, "Should this *guy be pruned out?"*

When I do not answer and stare bewilderedly at him, Jim Shotinger comes *to my rescue by explaining, "He means should we give David diuretics and* *mannitol to wring out his body fluids and shrink his brain," something we of-* *ten do when a patient has brain damage and the pressure within the head is ris-* *ing from internal swelling. Once I understand, I say, "No, the CT scan showed* *no evidence of increased pressure in the brain, and Mr. Ignatious does not need* *drying out." (I could never bring myself to call this "pruning.")*

Neither we nor the neurologists know precisely what provoked David Ignatious's lengthy seizure and subsequent coma. Of the several possibilities the simplest is an overdose of cocaine, but he might in addition have inadvertently injected too much insulin, or he could have had an ordinary stroke. None of these diagnoses, though, satisfactorily accounts for the impressive defect in his pons. Our responsibility is to keep him alive with the breathing machine and whatever else it takes so long as his brain might recover. We will have to be patient because the load of phenobarbital that was required to abort his convulsion might keep him unconscious for days. I ask the resident to measure the level of phenobarbital in his bloodstream so we'll know how long we have to wait.

Our second new patient is Katherine Khovenko, a twenty-four-year-old *woman who has been dialyzed three times a week for several years in one of San* *Francisco's best private medical facilities. Her kidney failure was attributed to* *chronic glomerulonephritis, a smoldering inflammatory process that destroys* *vital urine-forming structures within the kidneys. She was diagnosed when* *a young girl, a few weeks after she had had a bad sore throat. This sequence meant that her kidney disease was probably an after-effect of streptococcal ton-sillitis. (Rheumatic fever is another kind of devastating post-streptococcal com-plication.) According to her brother, she had been up and around the night be-fore he found her and called an ambulance. "She was just lying there," he said, "totally out of it." He added that she had been tearful and depressed since falling and injuring her left foot a week ago. He did not know why this had upset her so, but he speculated, "It might have been the last straw; she's gone through so much." After the accident, she saw her own doctor who prescribed a codeine-type painkiller and a powerful antidepressant.*

Since arriving in the ICU yesterday afternoon, Ms. Khovenko has not awakened in the slightest. All I can find when I examine her is deep coma with-out localizing neurologic abnormalities, plus a swollen black-and-blue area where her foot was injured. Her laboratory tests indicate chronic uremia. When we compare our values with those from the other hospital, however, they are nearly the same and do not explain her unconsciousness.

As with David Ignatious, we don't have a definite explanation for Kath-erine Khovenko's coma. We have to suspect that an overdose of drugs—prescription medicines in her case—might be involved. Perhaps she attempted suicide. At least her CT scan is normal. Again, we have no al-ternatives to the supportive care she is getting. We ask the kidney spe-cialists to see her because she will need dialysis tomorrow.

Then we see Maurice Wolf, who seemed to be worsening yesterday and had formed at least one abscess in his areas of pneumonia. The abdominal ultra-sonogram I had asked for revealed pockets of entrapped fluid in his belly, one of which was aspirated by directing a needle while using the sonographic images as a guide. The fluid contained many pus cells, but no microorganisms were sighted. Because of his probable intraabdominal infection, Ella Andrews started him on two more antibiotics. She appears to have hit it right because Mr. Wolf's fever promptly disappeared, and his chest x-ray looks a little better this morn-

ing. We wonder whether we are finally on the right track. "I think at last we're there," Ella says jovially.

Last but not least is Howard McVicker. After examining and hearing about him, I am persuaded to write in my note that he has just passed the "first really stable twenty-four hours he has had all month." The level of sedation was perfect, and he was wheeze-free all day and night. Another twenty-four hours like this and he'll be ready for transfer.

Molly Wolford takes me aside as soon as I return from x-ray rounds. "Hey, John, do you want to go in with us and buy some lottery tickets? A few lucky folks are going to win four million dollars; it might as well be us."

Lately there has been much talk and publicity about the lack of a winner in four consecutive California lotteries. Because the pot has accumulated so enormously, people are lined up at counters everywhere to buy tickets. I say, "Sure, how much?"

Molly answers, "Two dollars a share, but of course you can buy as many shares as you want."

I give her ten dollars, but add, "There's a special condition to this. You've got to help me convince Pauline to have some blood tests to check her thyroid function. I'll talk to her and fill out the forms. You reinforce what I say, and offer to draw the blood. She knows you're better at it than I am. I suspect she's hyperthyroid. What do you say?"

"It's a deal," she replies, slipping my ten into her pocket.

Saturday

When one of our medical residents overlooks a common disease in favor of a rare condition, we invoke the "zebra syndrome." It gets its whimsical name from the notion that medical students and young doctors in training are apt to interpret the sound of hoofbeats clopping down the street outside a high-powered academic institution by remarking, "Those must be zebras," never ordinary horses, reflecting the ivory tower preoccupation with things rare and exotic.

The zebra syndrome was hard at work a few months ago. I was attending in the medical ICU and saw a young Nicaraguan man who had been admitted the night before for severe headache, clouded memory, and stiff neck—textbook features of meningitis, always a life-threatening emergency. Analysis of his cerebrospinal fluid obtained by lumbar puncture (spinal tap) revealed chronic, not acute, meningitis, thus narrowing the field to a few diagnostic possibilities. But the radiology resident who read the patient's CT scan in the middle of the night saw a few shiny flecks in the patient's brain that he thought, erroneously, might be deposits of calcium. Based on this information, treatment was begun for "cysticercosis," a tapeworm infection that is endemic in Central America, which can involve the brain and cause calcifications. He was also treated for "herpes simplex," the cold-sore virus, which causes a devastating form of encephalitis, not quite what the patient had, and for *Listeria*, the "Cinderella of pathogenic bacteria," which usually causes acute meningitis, but which may display chronic features.

When I heard about the patient on ward rounds the next morning, I pointed out that these fanciful conditions smacked of zebras, and that everyone responsible had overlooked what the young man almost certainly did have and must be treated for at once: tuberculosis, the world's most common cause of chronic meningitis and unquestionably the leading diagnosis by far in someone from Nicaragua. Antituberculosis drugs were added, and four weeks later, the causative germ, *Mycobacterium tuberculosis*, grew from his cerebrospinal fluid. People tend to forget that common diseases are common, and rare diseases are rare. Jim Shotinger's three new patients last night and virtually all the others we have seen on ward rounds this month, with the notable exceptions of Clarissa Shafer and Ramon Bowsman, underscore this often forgotten principle.

The first of our three new patients is Quentin Green, a twenty-eight-year-old man with asthma and emphysema. Fourteen months ago he tested positive for HIV, but while on anti-HIV treatment, he has not had any AIDS-defining complications. Four days ago, he was admitted to one of SFGH's medical wards for diagnosis and treatment of two new problems: an abnormal tract (a "fistula") that had opened up next to his anus and was draining pus, and several swollen lymph nodes that had appeared in his groin, under his arms, and in his neck. A CT study revealed a huge spleen and many enlarged lymph nodes deep within his belly.

Yesterday, about noon, Mr. Green was taken to the operating room for excision of the fistula and biopsy of one of the enlarged nodes. As the procedure got under way, he began to wheeze, and his breathing became so labored the surgeon had to hurry the operation. After a brief stay in the postoperative recov-

ery room, where his asthma continued to worsen, Mr. Green was transferred to the medical ICU.

This morning his wheezing has improved but is still audible. His spleen and lymph nodes are so gigantic we take extra time to show them to all the medical students around. "Wow. Radical," one of them says. Mr. Green's chest x-rays have not changed in more than a year. All show that the upper halves of his lungs have disintegrated almost completely; the remaining gossamer network of strands that resemble cotton candy leave no doubt about the diagnosis of advanced emphysema. He is responding well to aggressive treatment for his asthma and should be ready to go back to the AIDS ward soon.

Quentin Green left the ICU that afternoon, and his asthma continued to improve. Microscopic examination of the specimens from his anal tract and lymph node revealed Kaposi's sarcoma, so chemotherapy was begun. He proves that, despite the availability of potent anti-HIV treatment, which usually delays markedly the onset of AIDS-defining complications, they can occur. Perhaps he didn't take his medications as rigorously as required.

The second new patient with HIV infection is Timothy Thomas, a forty-four-year-old unemployed man and regular drug user. He was brought to SFGH yesterday by friends who found him staggering around his hotel room, stammering unintelligibly. In the emergency room he was intubated, his stomach was washed out, and charcoal was instilled (as with Margarita Rojas, to bind with any unabsorbed drugs and prevent them from entering the bloodstream). Afterward, he was sent to the ICU, where he required machine-assisted breathing for a few hours. But he woke up nicely and was extubated about midnight. The toxicology laboratory reported that cocaine and a common type of antidepressant (tricyclic) drug were identified in the routine screening test of his urine.

When we visit Mr. Thomas, he is awake and alert but won't speak. In re-

sponse to my questions about what medicines he may have taken, he purses his lips and looks in the other direction. His lungs sound crackly, and he has a loud murmur over his big heart. His chest x-ray confirms that he has an enlarged heart and pulmonary edema. Diuretics to wring out his lungs are already working. He is ready for transfer, but we can't move him until he is seen by a psychiatrist.

About the time the psychiatrist arrives, so does Timothy Thomas's old medical record: he has tried to kill himself three times before. He is still incommunicative, and, because of this history, he is transferred to the SFGH inpatient psychiatry service. The record also points out that his heart murmur has been present since an episode of staphylococcal endo-carditis in the early 1990s.

We arrive outside the room of our third admission, Eleanor Dutour, just as her nurse shows up pushing a wheelchair to take her to the intermediate care unit. I put a hold on things to find out something about her. I learn that she is a thirty-six-year-old housewife whose husband brought her to SFGH yesterday evening after he got home from work and found her slumped in a chair, mumbling incoherently and breathing rapidly. He told the doctors that for the last few weeks his wife had been drinking ten to fifteen glasses of water a day and was getting up several times at night to urinate; also, she had lost five pounds despite a ravenous appetite. Although these are classic symptoms of diabetes mellitus, she had never been diagnosed as having it. Measurement of the level of sugar (glucose) in her blood now confirms she has it, and other tests indicate that she has moderately severe acidosis, a typical manifestation of out-of-control or, in Mrs. Dutour's example, new-onset disease. Acidosis also explains her depressed mental function and fast breathing. With intravenous fluids and insulin, her stupor vanished and her metabolic abnormalities corrected so quickly that Jim Shotinger has decided to transfer her.

I go in to say hello and good-bye. She is quivering with apprehension. As-

suming this is because she has just been told she has diabetes, I try to reassure her. She interrupts me to say, "I know all about diabetes because my younger sister has it. I am utterly terrified of having to inject myself with insulin once or twice a day. I've watched my sister do it, and it's unspeakable. I can't stand needles."

Eleanor Dutour is older than most persons are when the diagnosis of insulin-dependent diabetes mellitus is first made, but her symptoms are textbook pure. (It is better to use the terms "diabetes mellitus" or "sugar diabetes" instead of plain "diabetes" because, as Ramon Bowsman demonstrated on Day 19, there is another kind of diabetes, "diabetes insipidus.") Mrs. Dutour's stay at SFGH lasted only three days. She left in a much better mood, having been taught how to inject insulin under her skin, and finding out that exquisitely sharpened, tiny disposable needles are not as repugnant as she had expected them to be.

Surprising, and bad, news was telephoned to the ICU early this morning by the technician in the bacteriology laboratory: the specimens of Maurice Wolf's abdominal fluid and sputum are growing a "budding yeast," a potentially grievous development. Yeast, a kind of fungus that causes leavening of bread and fermentation of beer and wine, can certainly cause widespread, or "disseminated," infection. Even so, Mr. Wolf's lung disease is atypical and peritonitis is unusual. Moreover, yeasts are everywhere and turn up from time to time in cultures. Hence we're dubious, not of the findings but of their clinical significance. We have to make sure. If true, the prognosis is horrible; the infection will require treatment with an intravenous antibiotic, amphotericin, that stands a good chance of making him sicker than he already is. (Alternative anti-yeast medications are available, but amphotericin remains the drug of choice for disseminated infection.) We decide to obtain a CT scan of his abdomen and the lower part of his chest to learn more about what is going on in his belly and lungs, to recheck his abdominal fluid and sputum for yeasts, and to look for them in his urine, where they should be if he truly has widespread infection. We also ask the infectious disease experts to see him.

⬚

We hear next about David Ignatious, our patient who had a protracted seizure interrupted by anticonvulsant medications including phenobarbital. Since we saw him yesterday morning, he awakened unusually fast, probably because the level of phenobarbital in his blood proved to be much lower than expected. When I examine him, he appears to be ready for a trial to see if he can be extubated. A second CT study of his head, which the neurologists had requested, again shows the puzzling absence-of-cells abnormality within the pons. If we can safely extubate Mr. Ignatious, we will schedule an MR (magnetic resonance) examination in hopes of clarifying the nature of the lesion in the middle of his brain.

⬚

We learn that Katherine Khovenko, the second of the two new patients we saw yesterday with possible drug overdoses, is, unlike David Ignatious, not waking up. If anything, she is more deeply unconscious than before. The neurologists have consulted on Ms. Khovenko and join us in being unable to explain her coma. They suggest that we get an MR study of her brain if she does not start to improve. The nephrologists have also seen her and have scheduled her dialysis later this morning.

After ward rounds, Katherine Khovenko was dialyzed as planned, but cleansing her blood had no effect on her coma. I spoke on the phone with her personal physician, whom I remembered from years ago as one of our medical residents, and explained that though she was not waking up, everything else was stable. "Well, in that case, we'll take care of her in our ICU," he said. "We'll send an ambulance." Because there was no reason not to transfer her to her own doctor's hospital, she was trundled off that night, and we never heard what happened to her. That was a pity because her clinical picture was baffling—a profound coma that defied explanation—and I wanted to know what was going on in her body. Given our suspicious natures, we supposed she had overdosed on one of her medications. Yet nothing had been found on the screening test of her urine for toxic substances.

Last we see Howard McVicker, who continues to do well. Apart from a single episode of agitation and restlessness last night, but without the usual wheezing, he did fine. No beds are open in the intermediate care unit this morning; when one becomes available Mr. McVicker will be transferred there.

The wonderful thing about teaching medical residents, despite the inconsistencies and pitfalls, is that it really helps. Second-year medical residents have more expertise and sophistication than first-year residents. Third-year residents are even better: all three this month have impressive clinical maturity and confidence that complement their growing factual knowledge. Progress is evident during the year. Old residents move up a notch in July, when new residents start. Their lack of assurance and callowness in July contrast strikingly with their attitudes and behavior nine or ten months later, when I spend another rotation in the ICU.

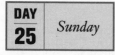

DAY 25 *Sunday*

The Etruscan shrew, the world's smallest mammal, breathes at the rate of 300 breaths per minute—six times faster than humans breathe, even during strenuous exercise. In relative amounts, this means that tiny shrews require six times more oxygen than vigorously exercising humans. Shrews, humans, and most other mammals breathe regularly at a fairly uniform rate and depth, but there are a few amazing exceptions. Elephant seals and sperm whales, for example, can chase underwater prey for up to two hours without breathing at all. The world's record for breath-holding, though, belongs to a reptile, the common lake turtle, *Trachemys scripta*. To avoid freezing in the winter time, it dives to the bottom of streams or small lakes, where it buries itself in the mud and holds its breath while hibernating from the fall to the spring—sometimes as long as six months!

As befits a process so fundamental to life, breathing is tightly controlled by nerve centers in the brain's most primitive hindpart. This is where messages are received from chemical and neural sensors that monitor the amount of oxygen and carbon dioxide in the bloodstream, the movement of respiratory muscles, and the behavior of the lungs.

238

The rate and depth of breathing are fine-tuned, usually to satisfy the body's metabolic demands for oxygen, but can be controlled for activities such as talking, whistling, or playing the trumpet. In the ICU we are almost always able to force air in and out of patients' lungs with a ventilator, whatever the cause of respiratory failure, but we doctors are not good at matching the amount of air we deliver to the body's needs of the moment. Margarita Rojas, for example, was overventilated and alkalosis resulted; this can be life-threatening, especially when the blood potassium level is low, as hers was. This morning we have the opposite condition, underventilation, and its dangerous accompaniment, acidosis.

It was inevitable and I knew it. Nevertheless, I am stunned and chagrined when Imelda Tuazon rushes up, grinning as usual, just after I walk into the ICU this morning to announce, "Claudia is back." And indeed she is. Claudia Jonson's stay in the intermediate care unit lasted only six days. Just after her arrival there, she seemed to improve; some even thought she opened and shut her eyes on command. She was dialyzed for what everyone hoped would be the last time, and then the dialysis catheter was removed. Two days ago, however, she developed pneumonia with fever and was started on antibiotics. Yesterday she became completely unresponsive, her oxygenation deteriorated, her blood pressure fell, and she developed severe acidosis. She was wheeled back to the ICU about midnight and was immediately started on a pressor medication to raise her blood pressure. She was also put back on a ventilator to raise her oxygen, lower her carbon dioxide, and correct her acidosis.

Just before we start rounds, a technician from the bacteriology laboratory calls to tell us that Ms. Jonson has two germs growing in each of two separate blood cultures: the particularly evil Pseudomonas aeruginosa, *and the always unwelcome* Staphylococcus epidermidis; Pseudomonas *is also growing from her sputum. Eight hours after returning to the unit, Ms. Jonson still requires a pressor agent, and, although she has been mechanically ventilated, her carbon dioxide has climbed even higher than it was when she arrived. This indicates that she is not being ventilated enough and explains why her acidosis has worsened. She opens her eyes when spoken to but doesn't turn her head toward the sound as she did before. Her morning chest x-ray reveals that the pneumonia has progressed. To top it off, her uremia is worsening.*

Dismayed as we are by the reappearance of all the formidable complications we had worked so hard to correct—deadly infection, uremia that requires dialysis, and respiratory failure needing ventilation—we decide to continue vigorous medical support for another twenty-four hours to give Claudia Jonson a chance to improve. Then we'll reevaluate the need for, and wisdom of, continuing the artificial measures that are keeping her alive. If her heart stops beating, though, we'll accept defeat and not try to restart it. I write a "do not resuscitate" order with a heavy heart; there is something so valiant and admirable in how she clings so resolutely to life. Is it just physiology doing its sterling work? Or does she really want to live?

Yesterday, I barely had a chance to see one of our new patients, Eleanor Dutour, as she was being transferred out of the unit. Today it happens again, though this time I get only a glimpse of a head and two arms protruding from the covers as the patient's bed wheels past us in the corridor. Ian Trent-Johnson was on duty last night and did his best to move the patient before I showed up, to spare me from getting involved. He just missed. Ian tells me that the vanishing bed is occupied by Yacoub Anastasafu, a fifty-two-year-old bus driver who was admitted to the unit yesterday evening with a brief but torrential gastrointestinal hemorrhage. His hematocrit, low at the outset, increased after six blood transfusions.

Because his condition stabilized rapidly, the projected endoscopy was deferred until later today. At seven this morning, Ian decided to move the pa-

tient, but no beds were available in the intermediate care unit. Had Mr. Anas-
tasafu actually left the unit before I arrived, my responsibility for him would
have ceased, and I might not even have heard about him. But now I feel com-
pelled to track him down in his new ward, check him over, and write a note
acknowledging his visit to the ICU. Without my note my department would
not be able to bill for his care, funds we desperately need to run the medical
service.

Next, we visit Maurice Wolf, our patient with a budding yeast growing in his
sputum and abdominal fluid. To verify their presence, a second pocket of fluid
in his belly and another specimen of sputum were aspirated and sent for culture.
Microscopic examination of a urine specimen revealed the same "budding
yeast," now from a third site. The infectious disease experts and we agree that
the evidence in favor of a widespread yeast infection is overwhelming, a grim
development.

Now that we know the worst about Maurice Wolf, we have to reevaluate the situation and decide what to do. Our options are to do nothing
and let him die, or to go all out by starting amphotericin and asking the
surgeons if he needs an operation on his abdomen to drain all the localized pockets of yeast. I learn from an infectious disease colleague that
his condition sounds hopeless, but one of the kidney consultants tells
me they have cured yeast peritonitis in a few patients receiving peritoneal dialysis—not exactly the same circumstance, but encouraging.
Mr. Wolf cannot tell us what he wants because he remains stuporous,
partly from sedation. Each time we try to hold back these medications,
he begins to squirm and look wretched and has to be resedated. We verify our impression that his social worker hasn't been able to locate any
family or friends, and we know that no one has visited him. Is Mr. Wolf
incurable and destined to die alone, or is there hope? I know he will die

without amphotericin, so I decide to start it, in the off-chance it will help, which we'll know in a few days.

◼

David Ignatious, with the mysterious hole in his pons, continues to recover nicely from his prolonged seizure and neurologic impairment. After we saw him yesterday, he did so well that he was extubated in the afternoon. We were thwarted in our desire to obtain an MR study of his brain because the scanner was fully booked and the next available slot is not until tomorrow. When we see him on rounds this morning, he is still sluggish and cannot tell us what happened to him, but because everything else is normal or close enough, it is easy to decide he can be transferred out of the ICU.

David Ignatious left the unit that afternoon and had his MR study the next day. We looked at the images out of curiosity (he was no longer our patient) and could see, once more, a region in the pons where nerve cells were invisible. The neuroradiologist could name several dire disorders that did *not* explain the disappearance, but she could not tell us precisely what caused it. I noticed she did not call the abnormality what to my jaded eye it had become: a classic "red herring," a seductive and distracting finding that proves at the end to have no clinical relevance. By now Mr. Ignatious has fully recovered. We learn that his seizures were caused by the big belt of cocaine he snorted just before he collapsed.

◼

Howard McVicker had another, for him, reasonably stable twenty-four hours. His temperature is resolutely normal, his asthma is the best we have seen it, and the sedation regimen is ideal. Try as I might, I cannot justify keeping him in the ICU any longer, so I transfer him to the intermediate care ward. He does not understand what is happening to him, but his wife is of two minds: she is overjoyed he has improved enough to leave the ICU, but she is petrified at de-

serting this familiar unit where she knows her husband gets outstanding care and where she is liked and welcomed.

After rounds, as planned, Mr. McVicker left the ICU, and a week later he was moved from the intermediate care unit to a medical ward. But his asthma relapsed again, and he went back to the ICU for a tracheotomy and second long stay; he finally left but then had to go back for a third visit. Neither his lungs nor his brain ever recovered their prehospitalization level of function. He died suddenly in one of the medical wards after ninety-eight days in SFGH, more than half of it spent in the ICU. Mrs. McVicker was working when it happened.

It takes me all morning to figure out that Jim Shotinger is dressed in green scrubs because he is on call today, and not Ella Andrews, whose turn it is. Jim says, "Ella left right after rounds on Friday to fly to New Orleans to be matron-of-honor in her medical school roommate's wedding. She's taking the red-eye back tonight." I wonder what kind of shape she will be in tomorrow when she is on call, but these three residents have done such a terrific job all month I cannot complain.

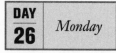

DAY 26 *Monday*

We live in a world of germs. Invisible microbes are everywhere: bacteria fill the crevices around our teeth, the canal of our intestines, and the hair follicles of our scalp and skin. Most of these microorganisms are harmless, but disease-producing bacteria are often mixed in and are constantly seeking ways into the body to cause infection. To withstand this unremitting onslaught, our bodies are magnificently equipped with an elaborate system of defenses that, first, prevents the entry of germs beyond certain barriers and, second, if some invaders should penetrate this outer perimeter of protection, quickly gobbles them up (technically "phagocytoses" them), employing vigilant scavenger cells that are continuously on patrol in the tissues and in the bloodstream. Reinforcements are provided by targeted antibodies and armed killer cells that collaborate to exterminate infectious agents. These mechanisms are not absolutely invincible though. As everyone has experienced, infections occur in healthy people, usually after they encounter a novel microorganism against which there is no immunologic protection, like a new variation of the common cold or this year's influenza virus.

But as Claudia Jonson and Maurice Wolf show today, and Fran-

244

cis Zohman and Howard McVicker demonstrated earlier this month, hospital-acquired infections are inevitable if patients stay in the ICU long enough. Illness debilitates natural and acquired defenses and leaves patients unable to respond to new infectious challenges or to keep old enemies at bay. In the ICU we make it easy for bacteria to enter a patient's body by routinely disrupting natural protective barriers with intravenous lines, intraarterial cannulas, bladder catheters, and endotracheal tubes. Lots of patients receive antibiotics, which kill many innocent commensal bacteria in the body and promote the growth of hostile antibiotic-resistant germs. We are repeatedly reminded that hospitals in general, and ICUs in particular, are dangerous places for sick people. That's another reason for moving patients out of the unit as fast as we can.

Our only new patient is Julius Upshaw, a forty-four-year-old man who describes himself as a panhandler, alcoholic, and occasional user of heroin. His trip to the ICU at 4:00 A.M. began with a series of medical misadventures that were set in motion about three weeks ago when he provoked a fight in a bar and got his left hand bitten; this was not a typical "CFI" (closed-fist injury), which occurs when bare knuckles chance upon exposed teeth, but was more an "MTI" (Mike Tyson injury), in which a body part finds itself within range of an angry mouth. The human mouth, especially when lacking dental care, abounds with potentially harmful bacteria. So human bites, unless properly tended, are much more apt to become infected than, say, dog bites. This happened to Mr. Upshaw, who came to SFGH eleven days ago with his left hand considerably swollen and the color of raw hamburger. The unhealed bite, now gaping from the swelling, exuded yellow-green pus. Sinister red streaks coursed up his arm and disappeared into the armpit: undeniable evidence of out-of-control infection spreading through the lymphatic channels.

He was hospitalized for treatment with intravenous antibiotics and local care of the wound, but the following day he developed marked tremulousness and delirium, typical features of withdrawal from alcohol. To control his shakes, he was heavily sedated. While nearly unconscious, he vomited and aspirated, which led to pneumonia in his right lung. Then his kidneys started to fail and caused a peculiar reaction known as the "nephrotic syndrome," in which the whole body swells grotesquely from retained fluid that accumulates everywhere, especially under the skin of the face, arms, and legs, and within the chest and abdominal cavities.

Finally, pulmonary edema ensued. Since he was having so much trouble breathing, the doctors on the ward attempted to aspirate the fluid from his right chest cavity to allow the lung on that side to function better. As happens in one out of ten patients having the procedure, the lung was punctured by the advancing needle and instantly collapsed. The surgeons quickly inserted a tube into his chest to reexpand the lung and mitigate a dire situation. But his respiratory failure persisted, and so he was transferred to us.

This morning he has a high temperature and responds to my questions only with moans and incoherent mumbles. His legs are edematous, and all his skin feels puffy. His new chest x-ray shows the pneumonia on the right has not changed much, but the pulmonary edema is worsening. His blood tests reveal progressive failure of his kidneys and ongoing acidosis. We can also predict confidently that everything is bound to worsen because, since his transfer here a few hours ago, his kidneys have virtually stopped producing urine.

Julius Upshaw is desperately ill, mainly from unexplained kidney disease. He needs dialysis right away, and the nurse-technician is already in his room setting it up. When the kidney consultants saw him for the first time several days ago, they suggested that his blood be tested for HIV infection, which can cause his kind of bizarre kidney disease. Although he prefers alcohol to heroin, he does use drugs intravenously, so an HIV serologic test is a good idea. But he has never been mentally alert and oriented enough to give consent for the "AIDS test," as required by California law. His course in the hospital has been aggravated by physician-induced ("iatrogenic") disease: oversedation led to his inhaling vomitus and developing aspiration pneumonia at the beginning, and his lung was accidentally punctured and collapsed yesterday—all-too-common accompaniments of medical ministrations.

■

We return to Claudia Jonson who, as usual, continues to tax our therapeutic prowess and our ethical sensibilities. We have been keeping her alive now for thirty-six hours, but the dose of pressor needed this morning is less than yesterday. Her body's poor oxygenation, carbon dioxide excess, and acidosis are a little better. There is no change in her mental state, however, and she intermittently twitches her head and left arm, a sign of more neurological impairment. Her left lung sounds less pus-filled than before, and her chest x-ray confirms that her pneumonia has improved slightly. The results of her laboratory tests indicate that her gathering uremia is slowly worsening, and her hematocrit is falling.

Now we have to make the decision we did not make yesterday morning, when we gave ourselves twenty-four more hours to see how Claudia Jonson would fare on the therapy that had been started when she was transferred. Today she is edging toward needing dialysis and blood transfusions, and we have to decide whether to embark on another long course of complex care in the ICU, with the huge investment that entails, in an essentially hopeless situation. I am convinced that she is never going to wake up. She has already spent most of the last four months in one ICU or another, with the result that she is now in and out of respiratory failure, requiring a ventilator, and in and out of kidney failure, requiring dialysis, and there is no reason to believe that her underlying lung disease and kidney disease will ever improve. Even more important is her mental condition, at best close to vegetative.

As we are discussing these issues, Dr. Richard Broderick comes by, having heard via the infallible SFGH grapevine that Ms. Jonson has been readmitted to the ICU over the weekend. To the delight of everyone, because he is so good at it, Dick has been head of the Ethics Committee for many years. He is joined by Molly Wolford, the head nurse, who knows Claudia well. We agree that we will continue treating her for the present episode of sepsis, which is improving, but that she is not a candidate for long-term dialysis or prolonged care in the ICU.

Another new and important episode occurred at six this morning: while drawing blood for Ms. Jonson's routine laboratory tests, her nurse, Betch Minerva, stuck her finger deeply with the needle she was using. Betch's first terror-stricken question was, "Is Claudia HIV-infected?" (The likelihood of transmitting HIV by a needle stick from an HIV-infected patient is low, 1 in 200 to 300, but unfortunately real: one nurse at SFGH has been infected that way, and there may be a second example.) The simple answer was we did not know. Ms. Jonson was originally hospitalized for injuries suffered in a fall, and all the subsequent horrendous complications seem indisputably related to underlying chronic diseases of her heart, lungs, and kidneys, not to HIV infection. We know Ms. Jonson is a transvestite, but we have no information about how sexually active she has been, or in what way. As far as we know, she did not abuse drugs. Betch immediately called our "AIDS Hotline" and was told that, in view of the uncertainty and pending a final answer, she should start taking zidovudine (AZT) at once. AZT, the first effective anti-HIV medication, reduces the risk of postexposure HIV infection by about eighty percent.[1] Experts now recommend adding one of the new anti-HIV drugs, called "protease inhibitors"; whether the combination is more efficacious than AZT alone is not yet known, but it is definitely worth a try.

The best way to lay the matter to rest would be to show that Ms. Jonson is not HIV-infected by testing her blood for the virus. Ordinarily we need her written informed consent, but under these circumstances we can legally perform an HIV test without consent—provided that a specimen of blood has already been obtained, that two attending physicians certify the results are indispensable, and that there is no breach of confidentiality. Since blood specimens are routinely held in the Clinical

Laboratory at SFGH, a sample was available and submitted for analysis that afternoon; I and the chief of medicine signed the required form. Had blood not been handy, we were prohibited by law from obtaining a specimen for HIV testing. In that case, Betch would have been forced to endure the side effects of AZT (at the least, fatigue and stomach distress) for at least a month. I think that is wrong.

Maurice Wolf has reached a clinical plateau. The budding yeast in the first samples of his sputum and peritoneal fluid are Candida albicans, *a ubiquitous fungus that commonly causes superficial infections of the skin (diaper rash) or internal membranes (oral thrush, vaginitis). Similar organisms are growing in the two newly submitted specimens from his lungs and belly, and also in his urine. This leaves no doubt about the diagnosis. He tolerated his first dose of amphotericin yesterday without the usual chills and fever. We are feeding him a high-caloric, protein-rich mixture through a tube positioned in his upper intestine. Despite the enriched diet, the concentration of protein in his bloodstream continues to fall, and he requires a blood transfusion every few days to keep his hematocrit at a decent value.*

The kind of disseminated candidal infection Maurice Wolf has is unusual except in patients who have marked depression of their defenses against infection, which he surely has. One glance at his emaciated body confirms that impression. Judging from his declining level of protein and his need for blood transfusions, his weakened condition is worsening, not improving. Moreover, the chances of eliminating the fungi from their pockets in his abdomen and the abscess in his lung, where yeast luxuriates, are slim. Did we make the right decision in starting to treat Mr. Wolf, or are we extending his agony as we are doing with Claudia Jonson? Even the pessimistic infectious disease consultant agrees that we have to try, for a while.

A common but underrated peril of medical management is pulmonary edema, the accumulation of extra fluid in the lungs. The lungs, however, are furnished with protective lymphatic pipelines designed to prevent pulmonary edema by removing fluid from the tissues as fast as it leaks into them, a fail-safe system that works beautifully—up to a point.

Medical students are taught that there are two different types of pulmonary edema: "cardiogenic," from heart failure of almost any cause; and "noncardiogenic," from injury to the delicate membranes that line the lungs' air sacs. This month, as happens every month, our residents have had to learn a third type of pulmonary edema, "iatrogenic," produced by well-meaning doctors who pump more fluid into a person's body, including their lungs, than the lymphatics can get rid of. Sometimes iatrogenic pulmonary edema is an inevitable consequence of an emergency resuscitation of someone who arrives at the hospital nearly dead (like Milton Trageer). It may be difficult to avoid when life-saving fluid must be poured into a patient with heart disease (like Edward Ramsey) or with lungs already damaged by infection (like Cesar Fonseca-Santos). But sometimes iatrogenic pulmonary edema is caused by careless physicians who believe that healthy lungs can accommodate any amount of fluid, which they cannot.

I admit that I am obsessed with the subject: all the housestaff know it. They even played a practical joke on me during ward rounds a few years ago. I was taken to see a patient who appeared totally hidden under the bed clothes. When I turned back the covers I was shocked to find a skeleton—the presumed result of restricting intravenous fluids and giving diuretics, which I had been preaching, to avoid pulmonary edema. My "patient" was nothing but bones! Yet I rest my case on twelve patients so far this month with iatrogenic pulmonary edema. And two more days to go.

"Code Blue," a frantic call for help, indicates that a patient (rarely a visitor or employee) has just died or is about to. A "code" usually starts with a nurse or aide discovering a patient who is not breathing or who has no pulse or blood pressure; the finder rushes to the nearest telephone and, using a restricted extension number, calls the hospital operator, who summons the Code Blue Team using a voice pager that announces the ward and room number of the victim. At SFGH, the third-year medical resident on call in the ICU (one of "my" residents this month) stops whatever he or she is doing and races off to take charge of the resuscitation attempt. That person will be joined by an anesthesiology resident, who rushes out of the operating room to intubate the patient, if indicated; by a second-year medical resident from the Coronary Care Unit, who helps with the electric shocking machine and drugs, which are often needed to restore an effective heartbeat and blood pressure; and by a respiratory therapist, who helps the patient breathe. One of the ICU nurses is on the team, because they are much more familiar with and skilled at cardiorespiratory emergencies than the ward nurses. All members of the Code Blue Team carry voice beepers when it is their turn to be on call.

Resuscitation still incorporates the basic A-B-Cs of emergency medicine: establish an Airway, support the Blood pressure, and maintain the Circulation. Doing all this involves rapidly escalating maneuvers to get the heart and lungs functioning again. Speed and proficiency count more during a "code" than in any other medical emergency. All incoming medical residents take a two-day course in advanced cardiac life support before they begin their first year of training, and they get updated at a one-day refresher session at the end of their second year. I, too, am obliged to attend refresher courses every two years. Concepts and procedures of resuscitation evolve quickly; drugs that were once mainstays of intervention become obsolete, and even techniques of compressing the heart through the chest change.

When I enter the ICU this morning I immediately notice turmoil in Room Six, where residents and nurses are shouldering their way in and out of a gathering of people milling around and blocking the doorway. Because nothing attracts a crowd like a Code Blue, I know what is going on and walk over to look through the window into the room. There is Ella Andrews on her knees; with her arms outstretched in front of her, one hand on top of the other, she straddles the body and rhythmically compresses the chest of a youngish-looking, disheveled man. The resident in anesthesiology, who has just performed the intubation, is pumping one hundred percent oxygen into the patient's lungs, while Marlyse Abbe, a respiratory therapist, readies a ventilator. The Coronary Care Unit resident places metal electrodes on the young man's chest to try to stimulate his heart to beat by firing an electric current into the muscle to jolt it into action. At first the patient is too acidotic for his inert heart to respond to external shocks, but this is quickly remedied by injections of an alkaline solution—sodium bicarbonate—and increased power in the bolts of electricity. Finally, a feeble pulse appears that is abetted by adrenaline and powerful pressor drugs. As Marlyse is connecting the patient to the ventilator, I see him making convulsive paroxysms of his arms and legs; these instantly stop when a muscle-paralyzing medicine is infused intravenously.

Half the crowd leaves, and I join the other half to learn what everyone else already knows: Kenneth Hines, a twenty-five-year-old vagrant, was brought to SFGH yesterday evening, wildly agitated from an overdosage of three kinds of antidepressants. After having his stomach washed out in the emergency room, he was admitted to the ICU for control of extreme excitement and tremulousness. Large amounts of three different sedatives barely relaxed him, and at about 7:30 this morning he started having seizures that continued despite jumbo doses of the usually effective anticonvulsive medications. Shortly afterward, while still convulsing, his heart stopped beating, and the Code Blue, which I strolled in on, was called.

When I finally get to examine Mr. Hines, he shows the effects of having just walked in and out of death's door. Nothing moves or reacts. His skin is bluish and cold, except over the left side of his chest and directly over his heart, where two patches of reddened skin are visible, each delimited by a fine line of charred flesh, showing exactly where the electrodes were placed that fired up his heart. I cannot hear his heart sounds over the burbles of the profuse secretions overflowing from his lungs into the air passages. His chest x-ray from this morning demonstrates the development of extensive densities in both lungs, which I interpret as either pulmonary edema or aspiration pneumonia, or probably both. The ventilator and extra oxygen are doing their job because his arterial oxygen, carbon dioxide, and acid-base values are now nearly normal. The levels of two of the three antidepressants he took are in the therapeutic range, but the amount of the third is greatly elevated and, as predicted by experts from the Poison Control Center, is rising fast.

The technique of massaging the heart by compressing it between the front part of the chest cage (breastbone and attached ribs) and the spine was described thirty-five years ago. Although introduced as a way to resuscitate hearts that had stopped beating in patients who were otherwise in good physical condition but had suffered heart attacks, cardiopulmonary resuscitation is now routinely performed on most hospitalized patients whose hearts or lungs stop working, *unless* they or their families have decided against it and the physician in charge has written an order that proscribes calling a Code Blue. Even so, cardiopulmonary resuscitation has often been performed on patients who have opted not to have it, though the frequency of this misstep is diminishing.

There is lively debate about whether cardiopulmonary resuscitation is a life-saving miracle or an exercise in futility. I am ambivalent, because every now and then a "code" works brilliantly; in between these magnificent rescues, though, it often causes more problems than it solves. A summary of results from more than one hundred medical centers around the world revealed that only fifteen percent of 26,000 patients who were resuscitated survived long enough to be discharged from the hospital; in addition, careful follow-up of 340 patients from a single hospital indicated that a mere five percent were alive one year after resuscitation.[1] Not unexpectedly, survival is poorest in patients who have unwitnessed cardiac or respiratory arrest (that is, they may have been without pulse or breathing for a long time), those on whom resuscitative efforts are prolonged, and those with serious underlying conditions, such as disseminated cancer, advanced cirrhosis of the liver, and end-stage heart or lung disease.

These dismal results differ strikingly from the outcome of resuscitations portrayed dramatically in three popular television programs, *ER*, *Chicago Hope*, and *Rescue 911*, in which seventy-five percent of the patients survived the immediate cardiorespiratory arrest and sixty-seven percent survived to hospital discharge. According to the authors of the analysis, who drew these conclusions, because millions of television viewers have been inculcated with misinformation, patients will expect similar miracles to happen to them. They and their families will be unable to make truly informed choices about resuscitation.[2]

Missing from these survival figures, not to mention the television programs, are the countless emotional and medical costs that derive from unsuccessful resuscitations that do not prevent death but postpone it a few days, or even several weeks or months. Also incalculable are the burdens of irreversible brain damage suffered during the period that the heart and lungs are unable to deliver enough oxygenated blood to the brain to keep it alive. Finally, the procedure frequently results in broken ribs, cracked breastbones, and traumatic injuries to nearby organs, the liver, the spleen, and even the heart itself. There is obviously no way now of telling what the outcome will be for Kenneth Hines. We have to keep supporting him to find out how much recovery he will make. It could be anywhere on the continuum from none to complete. If he does survive, we want to find out why he attempted to take the life we just gave back to him.

The other new patient is Sherwood Erlickson, a thirty-one-year-old commercial artist who sought help at SFGH yesterday for a troublesome cough coming from pneumonia in the upper part of his right lung. He was admitted to the ICU because his oxygenation was poor, and his cough was too feeble to get rid of the thick bloody sputum that welled up in his throat and made him gag. The resident tells us that Mr. Erlickson has HIV infection, but he cannot give any details because the patient has been so sluggish since admission. His lethargy suggested he might have meningitis complicating his pneumonia, so he has already had a spinal tap (lumbar puncture). The results are normal.

Sherwood Erlickson is another man with HIV infection and community-acquired pneumonia, a combination we are seeing so often. We do not know exactly what germ is causing the pneumonia, but he is being treated for the usual suspects and other less common bacteria. My colleagues and I at SFGH have the clinical impression that unusual microorganisms, such as *Pseudomonas aeruginosa*, which typically infects patients like Claudia Jonson while they are hospitalized, are becoming more prevalent and causing community-acquired pneumonia with increasing frequency in people with HIV infection. If the species of germs that inhabit San Franciscans have indeed changed, it could be explained by the widespread use by HIV-infected persons of preventive therapy against *Pneumocystis carinii* pneumonia with an antibiotic that suppresses common microbes, thus favoring the growth of less ordinary bacteria. Hence another clinical trade-off: the antibiotic suppresses pneumocystis and common bacteria, but when pneumonia does occur it is often caused by difficult-to-treat germs. As usual, the microbes are having the last word.

Next we go to see Julius Upshaw, our worrisome patient with rapidly progressive and undiagnosed kidney disease, who had five quarts of extra fluid removed during dialysis yesterday. This helped his pulmonary edema and improved his oxygenation, but not as much as we had hoped. When I examine him this morning he is continuously moaning, which makes it nearly impossible to hear sounds from his heart, lungs, and abdomen. I find no cause for his agony, but his groans are tormented. There is less edema in the skin and tissues of his legs by physical examination and also less in his lungs according to his morning's chest x-ray. His laboratory tests for uremia are about the same as yesterday's, and he produces only a trickle of urine. He will be dialyzed again today.

Maurice Wolf's monotonously stable course changed yesterday afternoon, but not for reasons we are proud of. While Ella Andrews, who looked a little bleary-eyed and conspicuously slow-footed yesterday morning after returning from her friend's wedding in New Orleans—the first time I have seen her other than vivacious—was helping the first-year resident direct a catheter over a wire that they inserted into one of the deep veins in Mr. Wolf's neck, the nurse reported that his blood pressure suddenly dropped, although just as quickly it returned to normal. The procedure continued, and successfully so. After looking at the routine post-placement chest x-ray, the on call resident in the x-ray department

*notified Ella that Maurice Wolf's right lung was partially collapsed—a com-
mon complication when the wire slips down through the tissues of the neck and
punctures the uppermost part of the lung. The surgeons promptly inserted a
tube into Mr. Wolf's chest, and his lung reexpanded fully. When we see him on
rounds this morning, nothing is different except for the presence of the tube and
its appended suction apparatus. I show the residents and students how to tell if
air is leaking through the tube. It is not, which means that the puncture site in
his lung has already closed, a good beginning. If we can get the tube out within
a day or two, this complication might not be as bad as it commonly is.*

*We visit Claudia Jonson and learn that she is continuing to improve. After Ella
took care of Mr. Wolf's collapsed lung yesterday, she started to wean Ms. Jonson from the ventilator. She has made such excellent progress that we switch
her to a system that forces her to breathe by herself. She still has pneumonia and
her shoulders and arms are continuing to twitch spontaneously, another alarming sign.*

Claudia Jonson is recovering nicely from pneumonia with septic shock
caused by *Pseudomonas aeruginosa*, which we knew had been in her lungs
a long time. We also know that *Pseudomonas* is nearly impossible to erad-
icate from chronically damaged lungs like hers, and is likely to recur.
The *Staphylococcus* that is circulating in her bloodstream undoubtedly aggravated her condition, but it should be curable because we have changed
her arterial and venous catheters and given her a powerful antibiotic.

A few hours after we saw her, Ms. Jonson was weaned from breathing
assistance without difficulty. That night she was moved to a medical
ward. Soon after her transfer, she became restless, and her twitches
spread to her whole body. When she started to have one intense con-
traction after another, which the neurologists interpreted as indicating
further brain damage from her recent episode of low blood pressure, intravenous morphine was started to eliminate any possible physical dis-

tress or mental anguish. She died comfortably soon afterward. Her blood test revealed she was HIV-negative, so Betch Minerva, who stuck her finger while drawing Ms. Jonson's blood, jubilantly stopped the AZT she had been taking to prevent possible transmission of HIV infection.

Ms. Jonson's total hospital bill, virtually all of it ICU expenses, must have been nearly a million dollars. She illustrates another paradox of life and death in the ICU that has been documented in other institutions: it costs much more, nearly twice as much, to die as to live.[3] When we look at the names of some of our other patients who died (Constancia Noe, Jean-Claude Lebrun, Cesar Fonseca-Santos, and Howard McVicker, for example) and check the length of their hospitalizations, we find that ICU care that ends in death at SFGH is also colossally expensive.

Of all our patients who died this month, Ms. Jonson was for me the most anguishing. Not because she died: that outcome was predictable when she returned to us in less than a week from the chronic-care facility she had been sent to. The collective clinical burden from her damaged brain, rotten lungs, and used-up kidneys was so punishing that she had to remain in an ICU to survive. Even there, though we are good at keeping critically ill patients alive, we cannot do it forever, and she was doomed. I think all of us in our heart of hearts knew that. What distressed me was that there was no room in our system for me to leave her alone and let her die peacefully. I was obliged by the rules to intervene, thus prolonging her misery and raising the cost. To this day I wonder what *she* would have wanted.

For a research-minded physician like myself, the most frustrating part of working in an ICU is the impossibility of ever knowing whether each of the many decisions I make is right or wrong. There's no doubt *why* a particular option was chosen or how it turned out, but there is no way of knowing what might have happened had I made a *different* decision. In contrast, a scientific experiment includes thoughtfully designed control studies to provide a clear explanation of the results, however they turn out. But there are no controls in the ICU. Once a decision is made to follow a pathway, that decision becomes irrevocable by preempting other paths that could have been taken. You can change your mind but cannot go back. Whether you succeed or fail, the route chosen is not going to be validated or invalidated by retrospectively analyzing it.[1]

Second-guessing seldom helps, but it is hard to avoid it on this, the last day of the month: Would Rosalie Larragasada be alive if we had given her umpteen more units of blood? What would have happened if we had kept Alexandra Papandreo in the ICU (and away from carrots) a few more days? Should we have acted aggressively and tried to save Eduardo Quetzel? How much neurologic improvement could Claudia

Jonson have made if we had kept her alive longer? The answers to these questions have no practical consequence, because all the patients are dead. But it is impossible not to indulge in this sort of hypothetical end game, and not to worry that the alternatives that were rejected might have proved better.

Our only new patient is Zachary Osborne, a thirty-eight-year-old legal secretary sporting a Salvador Dali mustache. He was diagnosed as having HIV infection six months ago, when he was evaluated for swollen glands. Since then he has been feeling fairly well and working regularly, until two days ago when he developed in rapid order, chills and fever, right-sided pleurisy, and cough that produced thick greenish sputum. He went to the AIDS Clinic but was referred to the emergency department by the nurse who discovered his temperature was 104.7° F. Because his chest x-ray showed extensive pneumonia and his arterial blood oxygen was marginal, he was admitted to a medical ward. Yesterday his blood cultures were reported positive for Streptococcus pneumoniae, *for which he had been treated. Without warning his oxygenation plunged, and he required intubation and transfer to us.*

This morning Mr. Osborne still has a fever, his oxygenation is reasonable while he is being ventilated, and his chest x-ray, which had worsened yesterday, is back to where it was when he was first seen. The cause of his sudden worsening is mysterious, yet he appears to be improving.

Zachary Osborne was extubated, transferred out of the ICU, and quickly discharged from the hospital. He highlights once again just how frequent community-acquired pneumonia is among patients with HIV infection. Perfectly healthy people like Barbara Rivera on Day 9 can be stricken with community-acquired pneumonia, but as our experience this month has emphasized, the risk is high in alcoholics and drug abusers, and higher still in HIV-infected people. Pneumonia generally looks the same and responds the same in HIV-infected as in noninfected patients, but there a few differences. Mr. Osborne illustrates one of them: in patients with HIV infection the causative germ of bacterial pneumonia is two or three times more likely to spill over into the bloodstream, where it can readily be identified in blood cultures, thus providing a quick way of making a definitive diagnosis; this is especially true for *S. pneumoniae.*

We visit Sherwood Erlickson, yet another patient with HIV infection and community-acquired pneumonia. The first-year resident tells us that, like Zachary Osborne's, both of Mr. Erlickson's blood cultures are positive for S. pneumoniae. *This morning, he is wider awake and coughing much better than yesterday. Now that we have a solid diagnosis, we stop the broad spectrum antibiotics and switch to penicillin, which is still the best treatment for susceptible* S. pneumoniae. *Because he no longer needs to be in the ICU, we'll transfer him to a medical ward where he will receive treatment a few more days before going home.*

After his release, Sherwood Erlickson did well but subsequently had two more admissions to SFGH for pneumonia, each time with the same germ, *S. pneumoniae,* in his blood cultures. He demonstrates another difference between HIV-infected and noninfected persons in the behavior of community-acquired pneumonia: HIV-associated pneumonias, unlike those in noninfected people, have a striking tendency to recur in exactly the same region of the lung and to be caused by the same strain of bacteria, after what should have been curative treatment.

Next we see Julius Upshaw, the patient with some sort of unusual kidney disease. He was dialyzed yesterday, which lessened his pulmonary edema and laboratory signs of uremia. Considerable abnormalities remain, however, and his mental confusion hasn't improved in the slightest. He needs to be dialyzed again, later today. Then we'll move him to the intermediate care unit. So far he hasn't had any visitors, but an ex-girlfriend keeps calling from Detroit. The nurses say she is deeply concerned.

Julius Upshaw required dialysis six more times while his kidney function steadily recovered and his pneumonia slowly cleared; the chest tube was removed one week after his transfer from the ICU. Accompanying this improvement his confusion and lethargy cleared up, and he consented to have the blood test for HIV infection. The day before he was discharged, the result came back positive, indicating that his kidney disorder was an unusual manifestation of HIV disease.

When we visit Kenneth Hines, the Code Blue survivor, we learn that Priscilla Breman, his nurse last night, was able to stop the stronger of the two pressor medications he has been on since his resuscitation. Imelda Tuazon, his nurse today, is steadily reducing the dosage of the other. It takes time and repeated calibration to wean patients from pressors. The nurse keeps turning down the rate of infusion until the blood pressure drops to an unacceptable level. Then she returns to the next higher, suitable dose, waits a while, and tries again. Over and over.

I tease Imelda, "Why don't you taper faster, or must we wait until Priscilla comes on tonight?"

Imelda smiles but fires back peevishly, "I know what I'm doing; you don't."

Priscilla and Imelda were applying a fundamental ICU principle: "You never know what will happen until you try and find out." Ian Trent-Johnson was guided by this same philosophy when he stopped the paralyzing drug Kenneth Hines was getting to prevent his violent muscular twitches. Would the spasms return? Now, four hours later, they have not. When I examine Mr. Hines I am disappointed that he remains unresponsive to all stimuli. His chest x-ray has cleared a bit, but a toxic level of the guilty antidepressant remains in his bloodstream.

At the time we saw him there was no doubt that Kenneth Hines's heart and lungs were beginning to improve. Even so, it was impossible to evaluate his neurologic function because the many medications we had given him to stop his seizures might have been clouding his brain—and he had lots of one of the antidepressants in his body.

As the drugs wore off, the pace of Mr. Hines's recovery accelerated. The next day the last pressor was withdrawn and he was extubated. On the fifth day, he woke up enough to be transferred to a medical ward; two days later he consented to an HIV test, which was positive. "It's no better than I deserve," he said. After twenty-seven days in the hospital, he was transferred to a convalescent hospital. Later, he was moved to a chronic psychiatric facility because of sporadic violence and the potential to harm himself and others. He remains institutionalized with residual speech and motor impairment and significant psychiatric disability.

With a mixture of relief and poignancy I walk with the residents down the hall to see my last regular patient of the month. (I am on-call until tomorrow morning but won't be seeing any new patients unless they pose special problems.) Maurice Wolf has at last improved. He continues to tolerate the amphotericin for his disseminated yeast infection, his temperature is normal, and his chest x-ray is definitely better. Nevertheless, we haven't yet weaned him from the ventilator, and he remains senseless and uncommunicative. His right lung has stayed fully expanded with the suction machine turned off, so we decide that it is safe to take the chest tube out.

The inkling of improvement that we observed on our last day was short-lived. Maurice Wolf's respiratory status would steadily deteriorate, and he would require more oxygen and assistance from the ventilator. Worse, after more than two weeks of amphotericin, he retained abundant yeast in his sputum and urine; I am sure they were thriving in the walled-off pockets of fluid in his abdomen. His kidneys were beginning to show the toxic effects of all the amphotericin he had received. Ten days after my month on duty, the attending physician who succeeded me in the ICU asked me to attend an Ethics Committee conference she had requested to discuss Mr. Wolf. As customary, Dr. Richard Broderick presided over the meeting of nurses, social workers, residents, and attending physicians who were, or in my case had been, caring for Mr. Wolf. We were on our own, because no family had been found and no friends had come to visit him.

Three things were obvious: his widespread yeast infection had not responded to treatment and could not be cured; he was becoming more and more uncomfortable; and he struck everyone as terrified each time a nurse, therapist, or physician came near him. As Molly Wolford reminded us, on Day 21, when he needed to have the endotracheal tube reinserted, he had said, "Only as long as there's a chance." No one—now—had any doubts: there was no chance. An infusion of morphine was started to ease the anxiety of his breathing difficulties, and Mr. Wolf was extubated. He died, at last truly undisturbed, the following day.

After ward rounds were over, I wrote fast in order to finish my notes earlier than usual. I had an important engagement at noon: I was to meet the three third-year residents and take them out for a valedictory lunch at a restaurant across from the hospital that specializes in nouvelle cuisine, Vietnam-style. I do this at the end of every month I attend in the ICU, but this time seemed different. It was more than the usual bond that develops from working together and dealing with the patients and their problems. We acknowledged that an affinity had grown among us that made this month special. But given the peripatetic habits of medical residents everywhere, it was not to last. Ella Andrews went off to Boston to be a psychiatrist. Ian Trent-Johnson became Chief Resident at the San Francisco Veterans Administration Hospital, and I have met him just once since that last day. Only Jim Shotinger stayed at SFGH, where he is on the faculty, and so I do see him once in a while when I return for another rotation as attending physician in the ICU.

The results of the blood tests I had cajoled from Pauline Victoria revealed a mildly overactive thyroid gland. The endocrinologists recommended treatment. They are right, but in a way it's too bad. A little spark of hyperthyroidism brightens a person up and appears to suit her.

The ICU consortium did not win the lottery.

ICUs exist to save seriously ill people, who otherwise are likely to die, and to restore them to lives of length and quality. Did we successfully attain this goal for the sixty patients we cared for this month? We had at least seven gratifying rescues: Edward Ramsey (gastrointestinal hemorrhage and heart attack), Jaime Aguinaldo (gastrointestinal hemorrhage and achalasia), Barbara Rivera (pneumonia complicated by unconsciousness from lack of oxygen), Margarita Rojas (chloroquine overdose), Virginia Powers (asthma), Susan Levine (asthma and chronic obstructive pulmonary disease), and Eleanor Dutour (onset of diabetes mellitus with delirium and acidosis). Two more patients, Bi-Ya Ng and Yacoub Anastasafu, responded quickly during their brief ICU admissions (gastrointestinal hemorrhage from peptic ulcers) and should do well. Without the ICU, all of these patients might well have died.

We unquestionably saved Adorna Brown (sickle cell anemia and morphine overdose), Charlotte Atkinson (esophageal hemorrhage and bulimia), Francis Zohman (asthma and chronic obstructive pulmonary disease), Milton Trageer (hypothermia and diabetic coma), and Ramon Bowsman (multiple seizures from low blood-sodium concentration). In view of the severity of their chronic medical or psychiatric conditions, however, the length and quality of their remaining lives are problematic. The same can be said of the twenty-seven alcoholics and hard-core drug users that we reclaimed from the acute complications of substance abuse. Experience has proven that their futures almost certainly will involve other life-threatening episodes until they ultimately kill themselves or quit using alcohol or drugs.

Kenneth Hines's life was restored after he nearly died from self-induced drug-related cardiac arrest. Yet he will spend the rest of his days in a facility for the mentally impaired because part of his brain did die while his heart was stopped. In a similar fashion we pulled Truman Caughey through several close calls related to his severe asthma and chronic obstructive pulmonary disease. Even so, he will never be the lively, happy man he once was because of the brain damage he suffered during his episodes of oxygen starvation. He, too, will live out his life in a nursing home.

We also had notable failures: Howard McVicker (asthma and chronic obstructive pulmonary disease), Constancia Noe (AIDS and pneumonia), Claudia Jonson (brain damage and lung and kidney failure), Jean-Claude Lebrun (AIDS and pneumocystis pneumonia), Peter Svandova (staphylococcal endocarditis and heroin abuse), Clarissa Shafer (AIDS and amoebic brain abscesses), Cesar Fonseca-Santos (streptococcal pneumonia), Alexandra Papandreo (asthma, chronic obstructive pulmonary disease, and aspiration of a piece of carrot), and Maurice Wolf (*Escherichia coli* pneumonia and widespread yeast infection). All of them died after long and unpleasant courses in the ICU. One patient, Jisoo Hong, shouldn't have been admitted at all.

Of note are the five patients who were transferred to the ICU for treatment of medical misadventures that occurred elsewhere: synthetic penicillin–induced anaphylactic shock, too much morphine, too much oxygen, drug-related kidney failure, and punctured lung. We caused our own share of complications to patients already in the unit: iatrogenic pulmonary edema in twelve patients and one punctured lung. None of these mishaps was fatal. Despite the injunction "First, do no harm," accidents are inherent in the practice of medicine, especially in the ICU. For example, thirty-one percent of patients enrolled in a prospective study of four hundred ICU admissions to two hospitals in France suffered complications.[1]

Altogether, fifteen of our sixty patients died in the hospital, either in the ICU or soon after we transferred them to a ward—a mortality rate of exactly twenty-five percent. One dead out of four seems exceedingly high, but it is within the eleven to twenty-nine percent range reported in a review of eight other top-notch medical centers.[2] Our death rate is at the upper end because of the vulnerable population that SFGH serves.

This furious medical activity cost a lot of money. During this particular twenty-eight-day period, our sixty patients spent a total of 230 days in the unit, an average stay of 3.8 days each. There was considerable variation, however, from only a few hours to twenty-five days. Although ICU expenses vary according to the severity of the patients' illness and the amount of physicians' fees, charges average close to $5,000 per day for each patient. This means that we ran up a medical ICU bill this month alone of about $1,150,000, or a little more than $19,000 per patient for stays averaging not quite four days. These huge sums are collected from various sources, depending on the patient's insurability: roughly thirty-five percent from Medicaid, fourteen percent from Medicare, ten percent from patients, ten percent from contracts, seven percent from Workers' Compensation, and the remainder, twenty-four percent, from the City and County of San Francisco. The majority of patients at SFGH, however, do not receive bills for the charges they have incurred, so they have no idea what the costs are for care in the ICU.

We must ask the obvious question: are these huge expenditures the way we should be spending our health dollars? Are ICUs clinically expedient or medically profligate? Their proliferation was based on the belief that they added a key element to the care of critically ill patients. But it has been difficult to provide rigorous scientific proof that clinical outcome is definitely improved. Several scoring systems have been developed to assess quality of life, functional status, and need for and use of medical services in general, though not necessarily the particular ones provided in critical care units. From the few studies that have been performed using these criteria, we learn that a high proportion of surviving ICU patients attain their prehospital functional level within six to twelve months after discharge,[2] but there are important exceptions to this finding. One year after admission to an ICU, mortality rates for patients with certain types of illnesses are extremely high: seventy-seven percent for patients with chronic obstructive pulmonary disease who require mechanical ventilation, eighty-seven percent for patients with malignancies of different organs and of blood, and ninety-seven percent for patients with malignancies who require mechanical ventilation after bone marrow transplantation. Thus some patients benefit from hospitalization in an ICU, whereas others do not; those easily identified patients in the latter category, a high percentage, should be offered the many infinitely more humane alternatives to ICU care.

The results of poll after poll have indicated that the majority of Americans want improvement in the way physicians provide medical care as the end of life nears. People favor the idea that physicians should help terminally ill patients, if they want it, either by assisting suicide through the prescription of a lethal dose of sedative medication or by euthanasia through the deliberate injection of a death-dealing substance. Doctors are invariably less enthusiastic than the general public about their would-be role as executioners, particularly in the prevailing legal climate that, except in Oregon, forbids it.

Attitudes, though, are changing. A survey of physicians published in 1998 documented the fact that physician-assisted death does occur, although on a limited scale, despite legal constraints, and that it would increase substantially if the constraints were removed.[3] Today, eleven percent of physicians acknowledge that under certain circumstances they are willing to assist suicide, seven percent are willing to administer a lethal injection, and six percent of physicians have already assisted death at least once. Furthermore, the number of physicians who would be willing to comply with requests for assisted suicide and euthanasia increases severalfold, to thirty-six percent and twenty-four percent, respectively, if these practices were to become legal. The survey also established, as well as could be ascertained, that the patients who requested assistance from their physicians were already close to death. The majority satisfied the four main criteria spelled out in the Oregon Death with Dignity Act, which permits physician-assisted suicide but not euthanasia: (1) the patient must be an adult with a consultant-confirmed terminal illness and a life expectancy of less than six months; (2) both a written and two oral requests must be made by the patient and must be voluntary; (3) the second oral request must be repeated at least fifteen days after the first, with an opportunity to rescind it; and (4) the physician must obtain a psychiatric evaluation if the patient's disorder causes impaired judgment.

And now, impressive information is beginning to come in concerning the first year's experience in Oregon, where the Death with Dignity Act survived two bitterly debated referendums and was implemented on October 27, 1997.[4] The first referendum to enact the bill was only narrowly approved, but the second to repeal it was rejected by sixty percent of the voters, presumably because the electorate had become better informed by the intervening court battle and public debate over the measure.

Terminally ill persons have not stampeded their doctors with demands for physician-assisted death, nor have droves of doctors rushed to end the lives of their suffering patients. Prescriptions for lethal medications were written for only twenty-three patients: fifteen died after taking the medications, six died from underlying illnesses, and two were alive when the data were compiled. Patients who requested and used a prescription for a lethal medication were concerned about loss of autonomy or control of bodily functions, but not about intractable pain; contrary to the fears of some, there was no indication that physician-assisted suicide was disproportionately chosen by or forced on terminally ill patients who were poor, uneducated, uninsured, or worried about financial loss.[5] Passage of the act may also have had unforeseen beneficial consequences related to the palliative treatment of dying patients: Oregon is third among the states in the rate of hospice admissions, among the top five in the per capita use of morphine for medical purposes, and has made available an innovative standardized order form that allows patients to reject intrusive ICU-type interventions designed to stave off death, such as tube feedings, antibiotics, and ventilators.

An analogous process, which was set in motion over twenty years ago, led to the broadly established ethical, legal, and medical consensus that now exists concerning patients' rights and physicians' obligations related to withholding and withdrawing life-sustaining therapy: that process included extensive public debate on a subject with immense personal relevance, catalyzed by key rulings from the United States and New Jersey Supreme Courts. Today it is widely understood and accepted that the patient (or surrogate for the patient) has the right to choose to start, stop, or refuse treatment. Under this public mandate, physicians must assist in making the decision—and respect it once made, although there are important legal differences among the fifty states.

Similar thoughtful deliberations about end-of-life care and the role of the ICU should be extended from Oregon to the rest of the country. We could start with a generally accepted principle: that patients who are irrefutably doomed to die within days or a few weeks, who can't be saved no matter what, should not be sent to the ICU. If "terminal illness" were formally and universally defined to denote a life-expectancy of six months or less, as it is in Oregon, patients with advanced malignancies or AIDS, end-stage heart, lung, or liver failure, and severe and progressive brain damage, would be denied ICU admission. This supports the premise that it is not worth causing more suffering and incurring extra expense to keep persons alive who are going to die soon anyway. Crucial to this argument is the existence of many alternatives to ICUs and hospitalization, including medical care at home, in hospices, or in nursing homes, all of which are less aggressive, less costly, and much more humane. This latter point cannot be emphasized too strongly, and this information needs to be broadcast to patients and their families. Such a policy would make it much easier than it is now to say no to an ICU admission in questionable situations; and, above all, it would avoid the cruel prolongation of dying that sometimes occurs. Doubts about the suitability of an ICU admission can easily be reconciled in consultation with critical-care experts or other specialists.

(A few exceptions to total restriction of ICU admissions for terminally ill patients are warranted: brief support following a palliative operation; an easily reversible short-lived complication; and an unintentional drug overdose, as happened to Adorna Brown.)

But the recommendation to exclude terminally ill patients from ICUs addresses only part of the problem. As illustrated by some of the patients in this book, it is easier to deny ICU care to dying patients, as we did for Rosalie Larragasada and Eduardo Quetzel, than to go through the prolonged agonies of stopping it once it has been started, as we finally did for Maurice Wolf but could never bring ourselves to do for Claudia Jonson. Because it is often impossible to predict clinical outcome early in the course of catastrophic illness, and because end-stage disease may sometimes be difficult to recognize during an acute complication, it is more likely that difficult decisions will have to be made after than before admission to an ICU. Even when we do not know at the beginning, after a few days of treatment the prognosis usually becomes much less ambiguous. If the issue is in doubt, though, treatment must continue, as with Howard McVicker.

The consensus in contemporary American medicine is that what the patient wants, if based on an informed decision and if feasible, is what the doctor should provide, a standard that should, in theory, obtain in the ICU. Critically ill patients, however, are often incapable of making an informed decision, so that their physicians must rely on family members or friends instead. Advance directives from the patient would help, assuming they address the relevant issues, but, as affirmed once again by our experience this month, advance directives are scarce. This makes it difficult to move patients who will no longer profit from ICU treatment out of the unit. Without explicit instructions from patients, and with families and lawyers looking over my shoulder, if life can be prolonged a bit, I have no choice but to struggle on even though the patients nearly always die relatively soon. Not only are these deaths intensely miserable, all the evidence (this month's accounting included) indicates they are extremely costly, which brings up an often overlooked but increasingly relevant fact: adhering to patients' wishes may conflict with the desire to limit the costs of medical care in the United States; in other words, the ethical principle of patient autonomy collides with that of maximum welfare, the policy of ensuring that limited resources realize the greatest possible benefit. Ten years ago, this was not a troublesome problem. Now, society seems progressively less willing to pay for "everything."

There are no easy answers to this dilemma. What the patient wants and what society thinks is warranted are often incongruent. One survey, which included both patients who had been treated in an ICU and survived and families of ICU patients who had died or could not be interviewed, found that seventy percent were totally willing to return to the unit to achieve even a month's survival; although many of the patients in the survey had poor functional status and/or inferior quality of life as determined by quantitative testing, only eight percent were unwilling to undergo intensive care again to achieve any prolongation of survival.[6] It should not come as a big surprise that patients or their surrogates preferred life, even one of meager quality and short duration, over death and were willing to endure another session in the ICU to stay alive. Woody Allen was speaking for these—and most—people, I believe, when he said, "It's not that I'm afraid of dying, I just don't want to be there when it happens."

The medical profession should take the lead in deciding what changes are needed in the ICU and in seeing that they are implemented. Several professional societies are wrestling with some of these issues. Whether or not they will solve all the problems remains to be seen. I am not optimistic, however, because one of the lessons we have learned over and over is that it is not easy to change the way physicians practice medicine.

This was confirmed, once again, by the results of a recently completed large clinical trial: doctors proved resistant to an elaborate campaign to improve patient-physician communication, including eliciting patient preferences for intensive care and planning for terminal illness.[7] For that reason, I think that nudging by the public will accelerate the process and ensure that it moves in the direction that society wants.

It is important for people who are clinging to life to fight for it, and the ICU provides the most favorable medical battlefield for winning the struggle. Yet we need to improve our understanding of how and why these battles are fought and what victories and losses result from them. Most of the truly remarkable improvements that have been made in ICU treatment since its beginnings nearly fifty years ago have been medical and technical. The ethical underpinnings of critical care have evolved much more slowly, and unresolved issues remain. Conditions have improved, and the future looks good, especially because people are beginning to decide what kinds of ICU treatment they want and don't want, and physicians are beginning to respond to these decisions. But this process has just started. Much more needs to be done to enlighten the public and to improve decision making. Fortunately, the advent of gentler and cheaper alternatives to ICU care for dying patients can ease part of the burden, but people need to know why those alternatives are to their advantage. The stories of the sixty patients whom we cared for one month in our ICU are meant to further our understanding about the marvels of critical care—as well as its imperfections—in hopes of introducing a few improvements that will strengthen the partnership between the medical profession and the society it serves. That, too, is worth fighting for.

NOTES

PROLOGUE

1. Dragsted, Lis, and Qvist, Jesper. 1992. Epidemiology of intensive care. *International Journal of Technology Assessment in Health Care* 8:395–407.

2. Callahan, Daniel. 1993. *The Troubled Dream of Life: Living with Mortality* (New York: Simon & Schuster), p. 33.

DAY 2

1. Zang, Edith A., and Wynder, Ernst L. 1996. Differences in lung cancer risks between men and women: Examination of the evidence. *Journal of the National Cancer Institute* 88:183–192.

2. Fleetwood, Janel, and Unger, Stephanie S. 1994. Institutional ethics committees and the shield of immunity. *Annals of Internal Medicine* 120:320–325.

3. Wackers, Ger L. 1994. Modern anaesthesiological principles for bulbar polio: Manual IPPR in the 1952 polio epidemic in Copenhagen. *Acta Anaesthiologica Scandinavica* 38:420–431.

DAY 4

1. It should be noted here that the situation has improved substantially. Medications to treat HIV infection, chiefly zidovudine (AZT, 1987), didanosine (ddl, 1991), and zalcitabine (ddC, 1992), have been available for several years; they helped a little, but their benefits were short-lived owing to the development of either toxic side effects or viral resistance. Contemporary treatment with so-called "highly active antiretroviral therapy," a combination of (usually) two of the older drugs with one or more new agents, especially the potent protease inhibitors, was tested from 1994 to 1995 and started to become widely used the next year. In 1997, nearly three quarters of the patients followed in the SFGH AIDS Program were receiving these medications, which have caused a spectacular reduction in mortality and in the frequency of HIV/AIDS-related infections and malignancies; overall, there has been a seventy-one percent decrease in the number of episodes of *P. carinii* pneumonia from 1994 to 1997. The events described in this book took place before such efficacious therapy was routine. Now we see far fewer patients with HIV and its complications in our ICU: a good example of medical progress. See Christopher Holtzer, D., et al. 1998. Decline in the rate of specific opportunistic infections at San Francisco General Hospital, 1994–1997. *Acquired Immunodeficiency Syndrome* 12:1931–1933.

2. Gaskell, Elizabeth C. 1966. *The Life of Charlotte Brontë* (1857) (London: Oxford University Press), pp. 317–319.

DAY 5

1. American Thoracic Society. 1991. Withholding and withdrawing life-sustaining therapy. *American Review of Respiratory Disease* 144:726–731.

DAY 8

1. Morris, D. Lynn, et al. 1985. Hemodynamic characteristics of patients with hypothermia due to occult infection and other causes. *Annals of Internal Medicine* 102:153–157.

DAY 9

1. Pasricha, Pankaj J., et al. 1995. Intrasphincteric botulinum toxin for the treatment of achalasia. *New England Journal of Medicine* 322:774–778.

DAY 13

1. Lehmann, Lisa S., et al. 1997. The effect of bedside case presentations on patients' perceptions of their medical care. *New England Journal of Medicine* 336:1150–1155.

DAY 15

1. Hook, Edward W. III, et al. 1983. Failure of intensive care unit support to influence mortality from pneumococcal bacteremia. *Journal of the American Medical Association* 249:1055–1057.
2. Oye, Robert K., and Bellamy, Paul E. 1991. Patterns of resource consumption in medical intensive care. *Chest* 99:685–689.

DAY 18

1. Nuland, Sherwin B. 1995. *How We Die: Reflections on Life's Final Chapter* (New York: Vintage Books), pp. 144–145.
2. Dr. Kevorkian was convicted in 1999 of second-degree murder and is serving a ten- to twenty-five-year sentence for killing a man who suffered from amyotrophic lateral sclerosis ("Lou Gehrig's disease") by intravenous injection, an event that was recorded and then televised. At his sentencing, the presiding judge said Dr. Kevorkian had no right to take the law into his own hands and told him, "Consider yourself stopped."
3. Humphry, Derek. 1992. *Final Exit: The Practicalities of Self-Deliverance and Assisted Suicide for the Dying* (New York: Hemlock Society), pp. 1–192.
4. Walters, Mark C., et al. 1996. Bone marrow transplantation for sickle cell disease. *New England Journal of Medicine* 335:369–376.

DAY 20

1. Blendon, Robert J., et al. 1992. Should physicians aid their patients in dying? The public perspective. *Journal of the American Medical Association* 267: 2658–2662.

DAY 22

1. Camus, Albert. 1991. *The Plague* (1947), trans. Stuart Gilbert (New York: Vintage International), pp. 96–97.

DAY 26

1. Centers for Disease Control and Prevention. 1995. Case control study of HIV seroconversion in health care workers after percutaneous exposure to HIV-infected blood—France, United Kingdom, and United States, January 1988–August 1994. *Morbidity and Mortality Weekly Report* 44:929–933.

DAY 27

1. Saklayen, Mohammad, et al. 1995. In-hospital cardiopulmonary resuscitation. Survival in 1 hospital and literature review. *Medicine* 74:163–175.
2. Diem, Susan J., et al. 1996. Cardiopulmonary resuscitation on television. Miracles and misinformation. *New England Journal of Medicine* 334:1578–1582.
3. Sage, William M., et al. 1986. Is intensive care worth it? An assessment of input and outcome for the critically ill. *Critical Care Medicine* 14:777–782.

DAY 28

1. Flick, Michael R. 1991. The due process of dying. *California Law Review* 79:1121–1167.

EPILOGUE

1. Giraud, Thierry, et al. 1993. Iatrogenic complications in adult intensive care units: A prospective two-center study. *Critical Care Medicine* 21:40–51.

2. Dragsted, Lis, and Qvist, Jesper. 1992. Epidemiology of intensive care. *International Journal of Technology Assessment in Health Care* 8:395–407.

3. Meier, Diane E., et al. 1998. A national survey of physician-assisted suicide and euthanasia in the United States. *New England Journal of Medicine* 338:1193–1201.

4. Chin, Arthur E., et al. 1999. Legalized physician-assisted suicide in Oregon—the first year's experience. *New England Journal of Medicine* 340:577–583.

5. Danis, Marion, et al. 1988. Patients' and families' preferences for medical intensive care. *Journal of the American Medical Association* 260:797–802.

6. SUPPORT Principal Investigators. 1995. A controlled trial to improve care for seriously ill hospitalized patients. The study to understand prognoses and preferences for outcomes and risks of treatments (SUPPORT). *Journal of the American Medical Association* 274:1591–1598.

ACKNOWLEDGMENTS This book went through several incarnations that were inspired by helpful comments from a number of my literary friends, Alice Adams, Virginia Crosby, Marie-Claude De Brunhoff, Carolyn Kizer, and Leonard Michaels. Frederick Hill and Lizbeth Hasse offered invaluable practical advice. Two physician friends, Dr. Robert Brody and Dr. John Beebe, made important contributions to medical accuracy and readability. I also consulted some of my colleagues at San Francisco General Hospital and elsewhere, Dr. John Cello, Dr. Henry F. Chambers, Dr. Charles Daley, Dr. Vincent Figeredo, Dr. J. Louise Gerberding, Ms. Mallory Hondorp, Dr. Laurence Huang, Dr. John Luce, and Dr. Warren Zapol, about information in their fields of expertise; everything that is written, however, is my responsibility, not theirs. My longtime associates, Dorothy Ladd and Erwin Yamasaki, helped retrieve information, and Aja Lipavsky reviewed the entire text. I also want to thank Howard Boyer, Robert Pack Browning, and Scott Norton at the University of California Press for their support and editorial assistance. Top credit, though, goes to my wife, Diane Johnson Murray, to whom this book is lovingly dedicated, for her constant literary oversight and criticism. Without her "intensive care" and encouragement, this project would have died long ago.

INDEX

Abbe, Marlyse, 252
achalasia, 95–96
acidosis, 234, 239
acute respiratory distress syndrome (ARDS), 196
advance directives, 221–22, 273
aging, inevitable health decline with, 71–72
Aguinaldo, Jaime, 84–85, 267; achalasia diagnosis for, 94–96; endoscopies of, 84, 85, 91
AIDS, 83, 151, 152; anaphylactic shock in patient with, 38–40; bacterial pneumonia in patients with, 102, 103, 176; death of patients with, 42–43, 58, 131, 136, 170, 175–76, 268; family informed of, contrary to patient's wishes, 15, 23–25, 34, 47; Kaposi's sarcoma accompanying, 57, 233; patient informed of diagnosis of, 56; pneumocystis pneumonia accompanying, 15, 31, 32, 38, 56, 57, 108–10, 124, 131, 136; SFGH as model

for treatment of, 37; tuberculosis among patients with, 219. *See also* HIV infection
alcohol: beneficial consumption of, 212–13; problems associated with excessive, 212; withdrawal from, 245–46
alcohol-abusing patients: with complications of cirrhosis, 12–13, 37–38, 61, 73–74, 86–87; gastrointestinal hemorrhaging in, 8–9, 37–38, 86–87, 126–27, 135; hypothermia in, 80–81; with infection related to human bite, 245–47; with injuries due to fall, 81–83; life support withheld from, 13–14, 16, 62–64, 86–87; not visited by husband, 98, 139; pneumonia in, 15, 80–81, 85–86, 152–53; requiring emergency dialysis, 203–4; with staphylococcal infections, 60–61, 77, 81; sudden death of, 116–17; with tuberculosis, 133–35. *See also* drug-abusing patients

alcoholic ketosis, 133
alkalosis, 239
Allen, Woody, 274
allergic reactions, to medications, 39–40
American Thoracic Society, on relieving pain accompanying dying, 53
amphotericin, 235, 241, 242, 263, 264
anaphylactic shock, 39–40
Anastasafu, Yacoub, 240–41, 267
Andrews, Ella, 1, 2, 264; accompanies attending physician, 16, 56, 102, 114; at Ethics Committee meeting, 210; attends friend's wedding, 243; busy on-call activities of, 17, 79, 91, 142, 173–74; calls for DNR for dying AIDS patient, 175–76; discusses patients with others, 19, 74–75, 79, 214; participates in accidental lung puncture, 256–57; resuscitation participation by, 252; starts antibiotics, 80, 81, 85, 229–30; talks with patients and their families, 56, 79, 80, 177; transfers patient to intermediate care, 199; weans patient from ventilator, 257
antibiotics, 151; anaphylactic shock due to, 38–40, 69, 77; bacteria resistant to, 152, 155, 218–19; effective against pneumonia, 151, 153–54; Medical Grand Rounds lecture on, 66–67; for severe asthma, 192–93; for staphylococcal infections, 99, 167; to prevent pneumocystis pneumonia, 102, 103; for yeast infection, 235, 241, 242, 263, 264
anticoagulants, 49, 50, 76, 161
arrest, patient under, 106–8
ascites, 116
asthma: adult-onset vs. classic, 88–89; agitation associated with, 10; combined with chronic obstructive pulmonary disease, 10, 22, 66, 89, 90, 186, 268; danger of sedation with, 41;

HIV-positive patient with, 232–33; mucus in lungs with, 75, 110–11, 196; reversibility of, 90; severe, life-threatening, 75–76, 192–93; sudden deterioration in patients with, 139, 163–64. *See also* chronic obstructive pulmonary disease
asthma-bronchitis-emphysema. *See* chronic obstructive pulmonary disease
Atkinson, Charlotte, 5–8, 267; bulimia of, 5, 21–22; psychiatric care for, 6, 21, 22; transfusing of, 6, 7, 16
attempted suicide: CPR for, 252–53, 255; by lupus patient, 182–84; psychiatric care with, 199–200, 234; repeated, by drug-abusing patient, 233–34; suspected in comatose patient with kidney failure, 229, 237
autonomy, patient, 24–25, 63, 274
autopsies, 164–65, 170–71
Avery, Shirley, 45–46, 47
AZT (zidovudine), 248, 249, 258

Babcock, Irwin, 83–84, 91, 93, 96–97, 113, 120
Balmuthia mandrillaris, 171
barium sulfate, liquid, 84
botulinum, 95
Bowsman, Ramon, 193–94, 267
Bradshaw, Sir William, 63
brain: *Balmuthia mandrillaris* infection of, 171; CT scans of, 9, 20, 29, 106, 112, 127–28, 143, 145, 170, 220, 227–28, 231; death of, 201–2; medications used to shrink, 228; metastases discovered in, 20, 21; oxygen needed by, 115; tumor discovered in, 9, 25
brain damage: inability to determine, due to sedation, 40–41, 70; patients left with, 214, 268; from subarachnoid hemorrhage, 193–94
breathing, 115–16, 238–39

breathing machines. *See* ventilators

Breman, Priscilla, 262

Broderick, Richard, 137, 264; on informing family of AIDS diagnosis against patient's wishes, 23–25; on medically induced craving for drugs, 186; on prolonging ICU care for neurologically impaired patient, 147, 210–11, 247–48; on treating substance-abusing patients, 204

bronchitis. *See* chronic obstructive pulmonary disease

bronchodilators, 33, 41

bronchoscopy, 75

Brontë, Anne, 43

Brown, Adorna, 184–86, 198, 267, 273

Brownstein, Clare, 82, 139

bulimia, 5, 21–22, 267

Califiano, Luigi, 102–3

Camus, Albert, 220

Candida albicans, 249

cannulas, x; jargon used with, 227; as source of infection, 189–90, 208

cardiogenic pulmonary edema, 250

cardiopulmonary resuscitation, 252–55

Carrera, Lois, 192, 208, 215–16

carrot, aspiration of, 164–65

Caughey, Truman, 9–12, 47, 268; extubation of, 40, 51–54, 206; improved condition of, 22, 48, 65–66; reduced mental functioning of, 40–41, 51, 214, 268; sedation of, 10, 11–12, 32; talks with mother of, 10–11, 22, 40, 51, 66; transferred out of and back into ICU, 77, 205–6, 214

cerebrospinal fluid, 145

Ceruti, Carol, 121

charting, 15–16

Cheyne-Stokes respiration, 168

Chiang, Wei-chi, 106–8

chloroquine, 183–84

Christian, Benjamin, 204–5, 216

chronic habitual suicide, 181

chronic obstructive pulmonary disease: asthma combined with, 10, 22, 66, 89, 90, 186, 268; pneumonia in patients with, 186, 192; problem of intubation with, 94; respiratory failure with, 9–10, 11, 12, 66, 70; smoking as related to, 10–11, 88, 89, 186, 192

cirrhosis: complications accompanying, 12–13, 37–38, 61, 74; gastrointestinal hemorrhaging with, 8–9, 37–38, 86–87, 126–27, 135

closed-fist injury (CFI), 245

clubbing of fingers, 86

cocaine, 195; diabetic man snorting, 227–28, 242; overdose of, 106–8. *See also* drug-abusing patients

Code Blue, 251–52; for asthmatic patient, 163–65; for attempted suicide, 252–53, 255

Constant, Ira, 3–4

coronary care units, xi, 27

costs: of health care for elderly, 30; of hospitalization for neurologically impaired patient with multiple complications, 72; of ICU care for dying patients, 258, 274; of "ICU Sisyphians," 162; of patient care in ICU, 269; of triple therapy for HIV infection, 120

coughing, with pneumonia, 111–12

Cramer, Jack, 18; asthma patient sedated and reconnected to ventilator by, 130; on patient's lack of understanding of English, 107; on sedation for intubated patient, 12, 96

CT (computed tomographic) scans, 114; of abdomen, 60, 61, 97, 147–49, 220, 232; of brain, 9, 20, 29, 106, 112, 127–28, 143, 145, 170, 220, 227–28, 231; as dangerous for critically ill patients, 97–98, 149, 196–97

cysticercosis, 231

Davies, Gertrude, 81–83, 91; CT scan for, 97–98; husband not visiting, 98, 139; improved condition of, 121, 128–29, 138–39; transferred to nursing home, 138–39; weaned from ventilator, 113, 121, 128–29

death: of AIDS patients, 42–43, 58, 131, 136, 170, 175–76, 268; of alcoholic patient with kidney failure, 117, 273; of alcoholic patients with cirrhosis complications, 13–14, 16, 61–64, 86–87, 273; bedside monitors turned off prior to, 14; brain, 201–2; definition of, 201; of drug-abusing patient with staphylococcal endocarditis, 169, 268; due to aspiration of piece of carrot, 163–65, 268; of elderly patient with multiple health problems, 44; in ICU, xii, 269; last-minute revival of energy before, 42–43; of morbidly obese patient, 158; of neurologically impaired patient with multiple complications, 258; of patient with *E. coli* pneumonia and yeast infection, 264, 268, 273; of patient with eye and brain disorder, 170–71, 268; of patients with asthma and chronic obstructive pulmonary disease, 163–65, 243, 268; relieving pain accompanying, 14, 43, 51, 52–53; of streptococcal pneumonia patient, 220–21, 268; sudden unforeseen, 117–18; tranquillity accompanying, 43–44; from withholding vs. withdrawing life support, 87–88, 273. *See also* end-of-life care

"death rattle," 3

Death with Dignity Act, Oregon, 182, 271–72

dementia, 2, 221

depression: in asthmatic patient, 122–23; suicidality scale for, 200

diabetes insipidus, 194

diabetes mellitus: cocaine-abusing patient with, 227–28; complications of, 204–5; new diagnosis of, 234–35

diabetic coma, 103–5, 125

diagnosis: from abnormality noticed in physical examination, 141–42; sense of smell as aiding, 125; therapy started before complete, 92–93; of tuberculosis, 134; zebra syndrome in, 231–32

dialysis: of comatose patient with kidney failure, 228, 229, 236; as dangerous for patient in shock, 117; of diabetic patient with complications, 205; emergency, for substance-abusing patient, 203–4; of neurologically impaired patient with multiple complications, 70, 71, 91, 98, 112, 147, 239; of patient with unusual kidney disease, 246, 256, 261, 262; as preventing diagnosis using sense of smell, 125

Directly Observed Therapy (DOT), 135

Doe, John, 106–8, 114

"do no harm," 68, 268

Do Not Resuscitate (DNR) order: alerting medical personnel of, 4–5; for dying AIDS patients, 110, 175–76; family's knowledge of, 64; for neurologically impaired patient with multiple complications, 240. *See also* end-of-life care

drug-abusing patients: in anaphylactic shock, 38–40; attempted suicide by, 233–34; with brain and eye disorder, 145–46; with complications of cirrhosis, 37–38; damaged superficial veins of, 38, 146; diabetic, seizure and coma in, 227–28; difficulties of treating, 118–20; with empyema, 85–86; with infection from human bite, 245–47; with pneumonia, 15, 85–86, 102–3, 144–45, 194–95; in police custody while hospitalized, 106–8;

requiring emergency dialysis, 203–4; in shock after using "dirty crank," 83–84; staphylococcal infections in, 60–61, 77, 142–44; with tuberculosis of heart, 223–25; unreliable in taking medications, 103, 105, 119, 120–21, 142–43. *See also* alcohol-abusing patients

drugs, illicit, 195. *See also* medications

Dudley, Paul, 207–8, 214, 220–22

durable powers of attorney, 221

Dutour, Eleanor, 234–35, 267

Edwards, Danny, 85–86

effusion, 223–24

elderly patients: aggressive care demanded by family of, 29–30; cost of lengthy hospital care for, 72; costs of health care for, 30; given aggressive treatment against family's wishes, 2–5

emboli, 143

emphysema. *See* chronic obstructive pulmonary disease

empyema, 85, 86

endocarditis, 143

end-of-life care: advance directives on, 221–22, 273; cost of, in ICU, 258; role of ICU in, 30, 272–74; verbal declarations on, 13, 43, 63, 109. *See also* Do Not Resuscitate (DNR) order; life support

endoscopy, 6

Erlickson, Sherwood, 255–56, 261

Escherichia coli, as cause of pneumonia, 154–55, 177, 217

esophageal hemorrhage, 5, 6–7, 8, 21–22, 62, 267

esophageal varices, 9, 62

ethical dilemmas: continued ICU care in absence of patient directives, 273–75; relieving pain with dying vs. hastening death, 52–53; withholding HIV infection therapy from drug addicts, 120–21; withholding vs. withdrawing life support, 87–88, 273. *See also* ethics committees

ethics committees, 24; on informing family of AIDS diagnosis, 23–25; meeting on neurologically impaired patient with multiple complications, 137, 147, 162–63, 202, 209–11; meeting on patient with *E. coli* pneumonia and yeast infection, 264. *See also* Broderick, Richard

euphemisms: for transferring patient due to lack of funds, 72; used at bedside of patients, 132

euthanasia, 52, 270, 271. *See also* physician-assisted suicide

extension posture, 29

extubation: mystique in timing of, 33, 169; by patients themselves, 33; risk of death with, 40, 51–54, 206. *See also* intubation

family: concentrating on bedside monitors of dying patient, 14; demanding aggressive care for family member, 29–30, 214; expressions of gratitude from, 16, 114; inability to discuss pain and death with, 10–11; informed of patient's AIDS, contrary to patient's wishes, 15, 23–25, 34, 47; not visiting patient, 98, 139, 177; patient intubated against wishes of, 2, 3–4

feces, odor of, 125–26

fever, 123

fibrin, 95

Final Exit (Humphry), 181

fingers, clubbing of, 86

Fiorelli, Alfredo, 60–61, 98–99; complications in, 118–19; left hospital against medical advice, 119; Morbidity and Mortality Conference (M & M) on, 78, 150; surgery for, 77, 78, 79–80, 91, 98

fistula, 232
Fonseca-Santos, Cesar, 152–53, 155, 173, 217, 250; abdominal problems of, 196, 206–7; conversations with brothers of, 177, 180, 187–88, 197, 207–8, 214, 220; daughter of, 152, 153, 167–68, 177, 220; death of, 220–21, 268; pulmonary edema in, 196, 250; worsening condition of, 166–68, 176–77, 187–88, 196, 213–14, 219–20
"free air" in abdomen, 148
Furukawa, Hanako, 29–30, 44

gastrointestinal hemorrhage: in alcohol cirrhotic patients, 8–9, 37–38, 86–87, 126–27, 135; diagnosing, 92; heart attack during, 49–51, 64–65, 76; homeless tubercular patient with, 133–35; in patient briefly in ICU, 240–41; in patient with esophageal disorder, 84; in patient with ulcers, 72–73
glomerulonephritis, 228
Grambling, Betty, 93–94
gram-negative organism, 172
Grand Rounds, 59, 66–67
Green, Quentin, 232–33
Guzman, Patrick, 13–14, 16, 19, 87

Haagsman, Herman, 105–6
Hantavirus, 151, 152
health care expenditures. *See* costs
health maintenance organizations, reduction of patient follow-up with, 106
heart: pacemaker for irregular beating of, 70; staphylococcal infection of, 142–44; tuberculosis of, 223–25; ventricular tachycardia of, 42
heart attack, during gastrointestinal hemorrhage, 49–51, 64–65, 76
Helicobacter pylori, cause of ulcers, 73

hematocrit, 9, 72
Hemlock Society, 181
hemoglobin, 115–16
hemorrhage: esophageal, 5, 6–7, 8, 21–22, 62, 267; subarachnoid, 193. *See also* gastrointestinal hemorrhage
Hensen, Jim, 167
hepatitis, 61
hepatorenal syndrome, 117
heroin, hospital admissions related to, 195. *See also* drug-abusing patients
herpes simplex, 232
Hines, Kenneth, 252–53, 255, 262–63, 268
Hippocrates, 3, 86
HIV infection, 151, 152; blood test for, 31, 83, 246, 248–49, 263; ethics of withholding therapy for, in drug addicts, 120–21; Kaposi's sarcoma as complication of, 232–33; kidney disorder as manifestation of, 262; needle stick with patient with possible, 248–49, 258; pneumonia in patients with, 102–3, 255–56, 260–61; triple therapy for, 120; tuberculosis among people with, 219, 223–25. *See also* AIDS
homeless patients: with complications of cirrhosis, 37, 47; with staphylococcal infection, 60–61; with tuberculosis, 133–35
Hong, Jisoo, 2, 268; extubated and transferred to ward, 5, 16, 19; intubated against family's wishes, 2, 3–4
Hope, Sir Matthew, 141
hospital: infections acquired in, 178–79, 189–90, 197–98, 208–9, 245; leaving, against medical advice, 81, 119, 134, 142–43, 224; pneumonia acquired in, 155; private, 72, 106
housestaff team, 2
Humphry, Derek, 181
hypothermia, 80, 81; in alcohol-abusing

patient with pneumonia, 80–81; in patient in diabetic coma, 103, 104

iatrogenic disease, 246
iatrogenic pulmonary edema, 250, 268
ICU psychosis, 41, 54–55
ICU Sisyphus, 162, 197, 209
ICU terror, 97
Ignatious, David, 227–28, 236, 242
infections: hospital-acquired, 155, 178–79, 189–90, 197–98, 208–9, 245; human body's defenses against, 244; related to human bite, 245–47
infectious diseases, 151–52. *See also specific diseases*
insulin, diabetic coma due to not taking, 104–5
intensive care units (ICUs): billing for care in, 241, 269; clientele of, xi-xii, 38, 46–47, 267; clinical outcomes of care in, 267–70; cost of care in, 258, 269, 273–74; death in, xii, 269; determining needed changes in, 274–75; French study of complications suffered while in, 269; history of, 25–27; irrevocability of treatment decisions in, 259–60; odors in, 125–26; oxygen focus of, 115–16; role of, in end-of-life care, 30, 272–73; survey of patients who survived care in, 274; typical scene in, ix-xi
internists, contrasted to surgeons, 7
intubation, 2–3; of AIDS patient with pneumocystis pneumonia, 109–10; of asthma patients, 10, 66, 88, 94, 197; avoided for dying AIDS patients, 124, 136, 175–76; counter to family's wishes, 2, 3–4; demanded by family of elderly patient, 29; of morbidly obese patient, 156, 158; problems with lengthy, 70, 94; sedatives needed with, 10, 11–12, 32, 40–41; to allow anesthetization, 85. *See also* extubation

Jerome, Jesse, 223–25
Joint Commission on Hospital Accreditation (JCAH), restraints policy required by, 179–80
Jonson, Claudia, 69–72, 268, 273; CT scan of, 112, 127–28; death of, 258; dialysis of, 70, 71, 91, 98, 112, 128, 147, 239; DNR order for, 240; Ethics Committee meeting on, 137, 147, 162–63, 202, 209–11; HIV test for, 248–49; improved condition of, 98, 112, 163, 172, 257; neurologic condition of, 70, 98, 112, 136–37, 147, 162–63, 172, 180, 188, 259–60; transferred out of and back into ICU, 188, 239–40, 257; worsening condition of, 90–91, 120, 247–48

Kaposi's sarcoma, 57, 233
Karsdorf, Henry, 194–95
Kevorkian, Jack, 181
Khovenko, Katherine, 228–29, 236–37
kidney disease: as aftereffect of streptococcal infection, 228–29; unusual, 246

Larragasada, Rosalie, 37–38, 47, 259; life support withheld from, 86–87, 273
Lebrun, Jean-Claude, 108–10; death of, 136, 268; improved condition of, 121–22, 130, 135–36
Levine, Susan, 186, 195–96, 267
life expectancy, life-style and, 74–75
life-styles: frustration with, of patients, 45–47, 204; life expectancy and, 74–75
life support: cardiac, 252–55; desired withdrawal of, with no hope for recovery, 211; patient rights regarding, 272; for sudden-death patients, 118; withholding vs. withdrawing, 87–88, 273. *See also* end-of-life care

life-sustaining therapy. *See* life support
Lightfoot, Wallace, 133–35, 219
Listeria, 232
liver cancer, 61, 63
liver failure, 13, 86
Liver Rounds, 99–100
living wills, 221
lung cancer, related to smoking, 20–21, 35
lung disease. *See* chronic obstructive pulmonary disease
lung punctures, 246–47, 256–57, 268
lupus, attempted suicide by patient with, 182–84

McVicker, Howard, 12, 273; abdominal problems of, 137–38, 147–49; confusion and restlessness in, 12, 179, 189; death of, 243, 268; drug-induced psychosis of, 41–42, 47, 54, 76–77, 97, 113; extubation of, 33, 78, 216–17; fever in, 112, 123, 128; as ICU Sisyphus, 162, 197, 209; improved condition of, 22–23, 32–33, 112–13, 173, 209, 222, 230, 237, 242–43; persistence of asthma in, 41, 66, 89–90, 217; reintubation of, 66, 197; sedation of, 12, 41, 78, 96; worsening condition of, 48, 66, 77–78
magnetic resonance (MR) imaging, 128, 236, 242
Martini, Hugh, 30–32, 47; improved condition of, 44–45, 48, 55, 56–57; informed of AIDS diagnosis, 56
medical errors, 268–69; anaphylactic shock due to, 38–40, 69, 77; lung punctures, 246–47, 256–57, 268; oversedation of patient, 246; pulmonary edema from excess intravenous fluids, 6, 83, 113, 208, 250
Medical Grand Rounds, 59, 66–67
medical residents. *See* residents
medical students, xii, 2, 28–29
medications: allergies to, 39–40; as al-
ways dangerous, 76–77; antituberculosis, Directly Observed Therapy for, 134–35; drug abusers as unreliable in taking, 103, 105, 119, 120–21, 142–43; patients with problems due to not taking, 102–5, 142–44; psychosis caused by, 41–42, 54, 76; sedative, used with intubation, 11–12, 40–41. *See also specific medications*
medicine, vocabulary in, 226–27
meningioma, 9
meningitis, 69, 231, 232
metastases, brain, 20, 21
methamphetamine, 195; popular names for, 60, 195; shock from injecting, 83–84
Mike Tyson injury (MTI), 245
Minerva, Betch, 111, 248, 258
mitochondria, 116
monitors, of dying patients, 14
Monroe, Albert, 38–40, 69, 77; damage to veins of, from intravenous drug usage, 38, 146; decline and death of, 58; improved condition of, 48, 57–58
Morbidity and Mortality Conferences (M & Ms), 68–69; on patient who aspirated piece of carrot, 165; on staph-infected patient in shock, 78, 150
Morning Report, 48
morphine: addiction to, 184–86; to relieve chest pain with pneumonia, 102; to relieve pain accompanying dying, 14, 43, 51, 52–53
Mycobacterium tuberculosis, 134, 219, 225, 232
myocardial infarction, 65
myxedema, 141

nephrologists, 91
nephrotic syndrome, 246
neuroradiologists, 114
Ng, Bi-Ya, 72–73, 267
Noe, Constancia, 14–15; death of, 42–43, 268; meetings with family of, 16,

23–25, 34, 47, 114; worsening condition of, 33–34
noncardiogenic pulmonary edema, 250
nurses, 18–19; needle stick in, 248–49, 258. *See also names of specific nurses*

obesity: as health risk, 156–57; morbid, patient with, 155–57
Oregon, physician-assisted suicide in, 182, 271–72
"orthopedic library," 166
Osborne, Zachary, 260–61
Osler, Sir William, 4
osteomyelitis, 38
osteoporosis, 72
oximeter, x
oxygen: brought into body by breathing, 115–16, 238–39; sensitivity to therapeutic use of, 157–58; smoking preventing prescribing of, 215–16

pacemaker, 70
pain, relieving, accompanying dying, 14, 43, 51, 52–53
panic attacks, 97
Papandreo, Alexandra, 88–89, 259; asthma of, 88–89, 97, 113, 122, 130; death of, 163–65, 217, 268; hematocrit of, 113, 130, 139; improved condition of, 122, 139, 146–47; panic attacks in, 97
paralytic ileus, 138
Pasteur, Louis, 152
patients: autonomy of, 24–25, 63, 274; housestaff team assigned to, 2; lifestyles of, 45–47, 204; rights of, regarding life support, 272; subliminal awareness of comatose or sedated, 137, 190; super-sick only, in ICU, 38, 267. *See also names of specific patients*
pericardium, 223
peristalsis, 76, 95, 138
peritonitis, 148; spontaneous bacterial, 37, 116

phagocytoses, 244
physician, attending, xii, 180
physician-assisted suicide: legislation on, 181–82, 271–72; physician opinion on, 270–71; public's desire for, 270; vs. relieving pain accompanying dying, 52–53
Pickwickian syndrome, 157
pityriasis rosea, 104
The Plague (Camus), 220
plasma, 49
pleural effusion, 224; lung puncture during procedure to relieve, 246
pleurisy, 152
Pneumocystis carinii, 15, 31, 38, 56, 57, 108, 109, 124, 256
pneumonia: in alcohol-abusing patients, 15, 80–81, 85–86, 152–53; antibiotics as effective against, 151, 153–54; aspiration, 195, 246; bacterial, in AIDS patients, 102, 103, 176; caused by *Eschericia coli*, 154–55, 177, 217; caused by *Pseudomonas aeruginosa*, 239, 255, 257; caused by *Streptococcal pneumoniae*, 153, 159, 216, 260, 261; diagnosing, 55, 92, 109; in drug-abusing patients, 15, 85–86, 102–3, 144–45, 194–95; empyema as complication of, 85–86; Group A streptococcal, 167, 176–77, 217, 220; in HIV-positive patients, 102–3, 255–56, 260–61; in HMO patient with respiratory distress, 105–6; hospital-acquired vs. community-acquired, 155; necessity of coughing with, 111–12; as "old person's friend," 4; in patients with chronic obstructive pulmonary disease, 186, 192; pneumocystis, in AIDS patients, 15, 31, 32, 38, 56, 57, 108–10, 124, 131, 136; transient losses of consciousness in patient with, 93–94, 111–12
police custody, patient in, 106–8

poliomyelitis, ICU developed for, 25–26

Powers, Virginia, 192–93, 267

prednisone, 31, 75, 89

private hospitals, 72, 106

Proctor, Lynn, 51–53

"pruning," 228

Pseudomonas aeruginosa, 239, 255, 257

psychiatric care: with attempted suicide, 199–200, 234; for bulimia, 21, 22

psychosis: drug-induced, 41–42, 54, 76–77; ICU, 41, 54–55

pulmonary edema, 6, 250; cardiogenic vs. noncardiogenic, 250; from excess intravenous fluid, 6, 83, 113, 127, 196, 208, 250; iatrogenic, 250, 268

Quetzel, Eduardo, 116–17, 259, 273

Ramsey, Edward, 49–51, 250, 267; heart attack diagnosis for, 64–65; improved condition of, 76

Regional Poison Control Center, 36–37

Rennes, Ralph, 73–75

Reposa, Natalie, 137

residents, xii, 2; clothing of, ix, 101–2; frustrated by life-styles of patients, 45–47, 204; increasing knowledge of, 237; obsessive physical activity by, 28–29. *See also names of specific residents*

respiratory failure, 11; AIDS patients admitted with, 30–31, 108–10; chronic, sensitivity to oxygen therapy with, 157–58; with chronic obstructive pulmonary disease, 9–10, 11, 12, 66, 70

respiratory therapists, ix, 19

Reston, Bart, 78, 79–80, 98

restraints, 179–80

resuscitation, 252; cardiopulmonary,
252–55; preventing inadvisable, 4–5. *See also* Do Not Resuscitate (DNR) order

rheumatic fever, 229

Rivera, Barbara, 93, 111–12, 267

Rojas, Margarita, 182–84, 199, 239, 267

San Francisco General Hospital (SFGH): clientele of, xiii, 36, 45–47; history of, 36–37; as teaching hospital, xiii; television in ICU rooms at, 190

Schwartz, Joseph, 80–81

scoliosis, 29

scrub suits, ix, 101

scurvy, 141

sedation: dangerous during asthmatic attack, 41; inability to determine neurologic functioning due to, 40–41, 70; required by intubated patients, 10, 11–12, 32, 40–41

septic shock, 84

Shafer, Clarissa, 145–46; bacterial and pathological reports on, 158–59, 170, 171, 173–74; CT scans of, 145, 170; death of, 170–71, 268; deteriorating condition of, 159, 169–70

Shawn, Rupert, 203–4

shock: anaphylactic, 39–40; blood flow with, 65; glucose drop with, 171; from injecting methamphetamines, 83–84; septic, 84; from widespread staphylococcal infection, 60–61

Shotinger, Jim, 1, 23, 28, 264–65; accompanies attending physician, 56, 158–59; at Ethics Committee meeting, 210; calls about intubating dying AIDS patient, 124, 131; deals with x-rays, 155, 186, 195; discusses patients with others, 74–75, 126, 173, 214, 228; fills in for Ella Andrews, 243; on-call activities of, 93, 178, 232;

starts medications, 31, 153, 156; talks with families of patients, 29, 54, 117, 144, 180, 187; transfers diabetic patient out of ICU, 234; weans patient from ventilator, 23, 129

shunt, 62

sickle cell anemia, 184–86

smallpox, 151

smell, diagnosis aided by, 125

smoking: chronic obstructive pulmonary disease related to, 10–11, 88, 89, 186, 192; lung cancer related to, 20–21, 35; prescribing oxygen prevented by, 215–16

Smythe, Marjorie, 149

"soft call," 93

Spencer, Richard, 61–64

spider angiomata, 74

spontaneous bacterial peritonitis (SBP), 37, 116

sputum induction, 55, 109

Stanley, Scott, 175–76

staphylococcal infections: antibiotics to treat, 99, 167; as complication for open-heart surgery, 160; of heart, 142–44; in hypothermic patient, 81; in neurologically impaired patient, 257; in substance-abusing patients, 60–61, 77, 81, 142–44; surgery to alleviate, 77, 78, 79–80, 98–99

Staphylococcus aureus, 77, 81, 99, 142, 143–44, 209

Staphylococcus epidermidis, 198, 208, 239

Stewart, Potter, 92

Stewart, W. H., 151

streptococcal infections: in diabetic patient, 205; Group A, 167, 220; possible aftereffects of, 229

Streptococcus pneumoniae, 153, 159, 216, 260, 261

Streptococcus pyogenes, 167, 217, 220

stroke, 92, 143–44

subarachnoid hemorrhage, 193

sugar diabetes. *See* diabetes mellitus

suicide, 181–82; chronic habitual, 181; physician-assisted, 52–53, 181–82, 271–72. *See also* attempted suicide

surgeons: achalasia therapy proposed by, 95; contrasted to internists, 7

surgery: for brain tumor, 9, 25; open-heart, 144, 160–61, 168; to alleviate staphylococcal infection, 77, 78, 79–80, 98–99; to stop hemorrhaging, 7–8

Svandova, Peter, 142–44, 168, 174, 217; death of, 169, 268; possible open-heart surgery for, 144, 160–61, 168

syphilis, rash with, 104

teaching sessions: Liver Rounds, 99–100; Medical Grand Rounds, 59, 66–67; Morbidity and Mortality Conferences (M & Ms), 68–69, 150, 165; Morning Report, 48; ward rounds, 132–33

television: in ICU rooms, 190; portrayal of CPR on, 254

terminal illness, 272–73. *See also* end-of-life care

Thomas, Timothy, 233–34

toxic shock syndrome, 167

tracheotomy, 70; for asthmatic patient with chronic obstructive pulmonary disease, 129–30, 138, 149, 216; for neurologically impaired patient, 70

Trageer, Milton, 103–5, 114, 250, 267

transplantation, organ, in Japan, 202

Trent-Johnson, Ian, 1, 28, 101–2, 264; accompanies attending physician, 56, 114; adjusts medications, 41, 262; arranges consultation, 138; at Ethics Committee meeting, 210; "code blue" participation by, 163, 164; discusses patients with others, 38, 66, 74–75, 109, 138, 173, 214; examines patient, 110; orders extubation of pneumonia patient, 169; researches streptococcal infection, 166–67, 173; supervises catheter replacement, 190; talks with patients and their families, 43, 62–63, 169, 187, 207–8; transfers patient out of ICU, 240–41

troponin, 49

Tuazon, Imelda, 16, 18; on condition of neurologically impaired patient, 163, 239; on need to sedate intubated patient, 10, 12, 32; reduces patient medications, 262; talks with family of dying streptococcal pneumonia patient, 177, 187

tuberculosis: as cause of meningitis, 232; Directly Observed Therapy for, 134–35; of heart, 223–25; homeless patient with, 133–35, 219; resurgence of, 151, 152, 218–19, 225

Tutupoa, Marshall, 155–58, 217

Twist, Adrian, 95

ulcers, 72–73, 86

Upshaw, Julius, 245–47, 256, 261–62

uremia, 70, 71, 90–91, 125

urethra, 80

vegetative state, 202

ventilators, x, 26, 239. *See also* extubation; intubation

ventricular tachycardia, 42

Victoria, Pauline: hyperthyroidism of, 179, 230, 265; interacts with dying AIDS patient and family, 24, 34, 42, 114; updates confused patient, 179

Viragio, Elisabeth, 49–50

vitamin K, 49

vocabulary, medical, 226–27

Vysinsky, Gyula, 19–21, 35

Walter (cat), 17, 100, 124, 140, 175, 191–92, 217

ward rounds: change in style and for-

mality of, 132–33; Liver Rounds, 99–100; Medical Grand Rounds, 59, 66–67

Washington, Althanette, 8–9, 25

Williams, Jesse, 144–45, 159–60, 169

Wolf, Maurice, 154–55, 171–72, 217; death of, 264, 268, 273; improved condition of, 188–89, 209, 215, 229–30, 263; punctured lung of, 256–57; transfusion of, 177–78, 189; worsening pneumonia in, 189, 198–99, 215, 222; yeast infection in, 235–36, 241–42, 249, 263, 264

Wolford, Molly, 18, 222, 230, 248; at transfer of patient to rehab center, 264; communicates about medication-induced anaphylactic shock, 39–40; on patient's directive regarding intubation, 264; turns off bedside monitor of dying patient, 14

"The Wonderful One-Hoss Shay" (Holmes), 71

Wu, Andrew, 107–8

x-rays, missing, 186–87

yeast infection, 235–36, 241–42, 249, 263

Younger, Amos, 126–27, 135

zebra syndrome, 231–32

zidovudine (AZT), 248, 249, 258

Zohman, Francis, 75–76, 217, 267; clearing of obstructed lung of, 75, 110–11; depression in, 122–23; hospital-acquired infection in, 178–79, 189–90, 197–98, 208–9; improved condition of, 89, 149, 161–62, 172–73, 216; intubation of, 94, 129; tracheotomy for, 129–30, 138, 149, 216; transferred out of and back into ICU, 77, 89, 222–23

Designer:	Nicole Hayward
Compositor:	G&S Typesetters
Text:	10/15 Janson
Display:	Akzidenz Grotesk, Scala
Printer and binder:	Edwards Brothers

62

362.174   Murray, John F. (John
MUR   Frederic),
             1927-

        Intensive care.